Tian yow Tsong

Johns Hopkins University

School of Medicine

6-12-79

Membrane Proteins
and their Interactions
with Lipids

Membrane Proteins

EDITOR
RODERICK A. CAPALDI

Institute of Molecular Biology
University of Oregon
Eugene, Oregon

Membrane Proteins and their Interactions with Lipids

edited by

RODERICK A. CAPALDI

Institute of Molecular Biology
University of Oregon
Eugene, Oregon

MARCEL DEKKER, INC.   New York and Basel

Library of Congress Cataloging in Publication Data
Main entry under title:

Membrane proteins and their interactions with lipids.

  (Membrane proteins ; v. 1)
  Includes bibliographies and indexes.
  1. Membrane proteins. 2. Bilayer lipid membranes.
3. Biochemorphology. I. Capaldi, Roderick A. II. Series. [DNLM: 1. Membrane proteins. 2. Membrane
lipids. 3. Biological transport. W1 ME8935 v. 1 /
QU55 M533]
QP552.M44M45   574.8'75   76-58609
ISBN 0-8247-6595-8

MARCEL DEKKER, INC.

270 Madison Avenue, New York, New York 10016

Current printing (last digit):
10 9 8 7 6 5 4 3 2 1

PRINTED IN THE UNITED STATES OF AMERICA

Membrane proteins are involved in many of the important functions of cells including energy transduction, transport of substances in and out of a cell or organelle, lipid metabolism, hormonal action, and cellular control. Procedures for isolating membrane proteins in an active form are continually being refined. As a result, more and more functionally important membrane proteins are being isolated and a vast body of literature on the structure and function of these proteins is accumulating. Studies of membrane proteins are published in journals of hematology, virology, bacteriology, and immunology as well as in journals of biology and biochemistry. Consequently, it becomes progressively more difficult to keep up with advances in this diverse area of research. The more diverse a field becomes, the more important it is to have available recent reviews on specific aspects of that area of research.

The aim of this series is to provide a forum for discussion of advances in our understanding of both the structure and function of membrane proteins. As far as possible, individual volumes will concentrate on areas in which significant progress is being made such as in protein-lipid interactions, energy transduction, and hormone-receptor interactions. In this way the volumes shall be an important reference source for advanced students interested in membrane-related phenomena as well as researchers in the selected areas.

Roderick A. Capaldi

The field of membrane structure has made rapid strides in the last few years. Prior to about 1970 the unit membrane model in which the protein was restricted to the surfaces of a lipid bilayer was dominant. More recently it has become obvious that many proteins penetrate into and even completely through the lipid bilayer. This raises several questions about the structure of membrane proteins and their interaction with lipids, such as: what are the structural features of a protein which allow it to be at least partly buried in an essentially hydrocarbon medium (inside the bilayer); what types of forces are involved in lipid protein interactions; what role if any do lipids play in the functioning of enzymes or transport proteins which are embedded in the membrane?

The available information bearing on these three questions is reviewed in this volume. The structural features of membrane proteins are reviewed in Chapters 1 and 2. The interaction of proteins and lipids is considered in two chapters, the association of proteins with lipids in membranes and serum lipoproteins being compared in Chapter 2 while a comprehensive review of the properties of lipids and their association with proteins is presented in Chapter 3. The properties of the proteins in Semliki Forest virus and the interaction of these proteins with lipids and detergents are also reviewed. Finally, chapters on the Ca^{2+} ATPase and Na^+-K^+ ATPase discuss the structure and function of these proteins and examine the role that lipids play in the functioning of these transport proteins.

I am grateful to the authors for their contributions, and I would also like to express my gratitude to the staff of Marcel Dekker, Inc. for their help in the production of this book.

Roderick A. Capaldi

CONTENTS

CONTRIBUTORS

RONALD E. BARNETT[*]   Department of Chemistry, University of Minnesota, Minneapolis, Minnesota

RONALD J. BASKIN   Department of Zoology, University of California, Davis, California

RODERICK A. CAPALDI   Institute of Molecular Biology, University of Oregon, Eugene, Oregon

HENRIK GAROFF   European Molecular Biology Laboratory, Heidelberg, Federal Republic of Germany

ARI HELENIUS   European Molecular Biology Laboratory, Heidelberg, Federal Republic of Germany

RICHARD L. JACKSON   Department of Medicine, Baylor College of Medicine, and the Methodist Hospital, Houston Texas

GIORGIO LENAZ   Istituto di Biochimica, Facoltà di Medicina e Chirurgia, University of Ancona, Italy

JERE P. SEGREST   Comprehensive Cancer Center, Department of Pathology, Birmingham Medical Center, Birmingham, Alabama

KAI SIMONS   European Molecular Biology Laboratory, Heidelberg, Federal Republic of Germany

_____

[*] Current affiliation: Department of Biochemistry and Nutrition, Virginia Polytechnic Institute and State University, Blacksburg, Virginia.

Chapter 1

THE STRUCTURAL PROPERTIES OF MEMBRANE PROTEINS

Roderick A. Capaldi

Institute of Molecular Biology
University of Oregon
Eugene, Oregon

I. INTRODUCTION

Considerable progress has been made in recent years in understanding the structure and functioning of membrane proteins. Important components that transport substrates or ions into and out of the cell, and also proteins that are involved in the biosynthesis and degradation of lipids, in oxidative phosphorylation and in photosynthesis, and that act as receptors and effectors of cellular control have been identified as membrane-bound. This review is written with the question in mind, are membrane proteins different structurally from nonmembrane proteins?

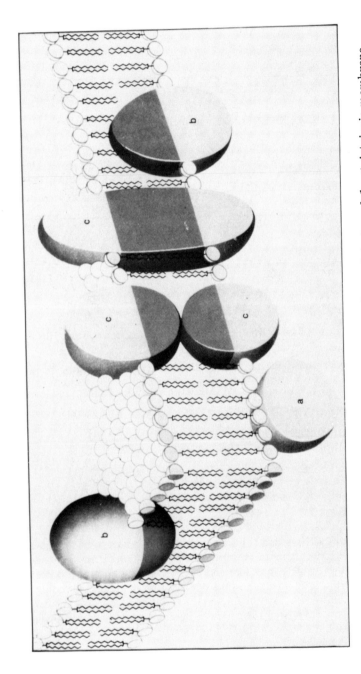

FIG. 1 A schematic representation of the association of (a) extrinsic and (b, c) intrinsic membrane proteins with the lipid bilayer in membranes. (Reprinted from Sci. Am. March, 1974, with the kind permission of W. H. Freeman & Company, publishers.)

II. MEMBRANE MODELS

Implicit in all recent pictures of membrane structure is the idea that the lipid in membranes is in the form of a bilayer with proteins sitting on the surface or penetrating the lipid bilayer wholly or partially (Fig. 1). Proteins to be discussed in this review are those that are tightly associated with the lipids and an integral part of the membrane continuum. In recent terminology, these would be intrinsic [1, 2], or integral [3], membrane proteins. (I shall consider the classification of membrane proteins into intrinsic and extrinsic proteins later.)

III. ISOLATION OF MEMBRANE PROTEINS WITH LIPOPHILIC SOLVENTS

Intrinsic membrane proteins can be isolated only after the membrane continuum has been disrupted. A variety of organic solvents have been used to dissolve membranes, including 35% aqueous pyridine [4], lithium diiodosalicylate [5], chloroform-methanol [6], phenol [7], n-butanol [8], and chloroethanol [9]. These methods solubilize protein but for the most part in a denatured form suitable for analyzing primary structure only. Proteins that dissolve in chloroform-methanol (2:1 v/v) are generally called proteolipids [10]. Proteins soluble in this organic solvent mixture were isolated originally from myelin [11, 12] but have also been extracted from mitochondrial membranes [13-15], sarcoplasmic reticulum [16], and nerve endings [17-19]. Mitochondrial proteolipids have been identified as polypeptide components of cytochrome oxidase [20] and the oligomycin-sensitive ATPase [14]. These are all synthesized within mitochondria and are coded for by mitochondrial DNA [20, 21]. The sarcoplasmic reticulum proteolipid is associated with the Ca^{2+}-Mg^{2+} ATPase [16] and has been implicated recently in calcium translocation. Proteolipids from nerve endings may be the receptor for acetylcholine or at least a part of a receptor complex. A chloroform-methanol soluble fraction from nerve endings apparently binds acetylcholine in a way that is inhibited by α-bungarotoxin [17]. When this proteolipid fraction is incorporated into black lipid membranes, it demonstrates acetylcholine-stimulated conductivity of ions through the bilayer [18, 19].

Proteolipids are among the most hydrophobic proteins yet characterized; they contain a high percentage of apolar amino acids (Table 1). The myelin proteolipids and sarcoplasmic reticulum proteolipids have in addition covalently bound fatty acids (3% by weight of the myelin proteolipid [10, 16]), which would be expected to enhance their solubility in organic solvent. Yet some, at least, of these proteins can be obtained in a water-soluble form. Tennenbaum and Folch-Pi [22] were able to convert the proteolipid of myelin into a water-soluble form by dialyzing the protein suspended in organic solvent against dialysate of increasing water content. The aqueous solubility of these most hydrophobic of intrinsic membrane proteins is

TABLE 1

Percentage of Apolar Amino Acids in Proteolipids

	Folch-Lees[a] proteolipid (bovine)	Subunit I, cytochrome oxidase[b]	Proteolipid of the oligomycin-sensitive ATPase[c]
Lys	4.8	4.4	3.4
His	2.3	2.1	trace
Arg	3.0	2.3	1.5
Asp	4.4	7.8	4.7
Thr	8.6	5.1	4.6
Ser	6.7	7.2	6.9
Glu	6.6	5.9	3.1
Total in mole %	36.4	34.8	24.2
Pro	2.3	4.3	3.1
Gly	11.0	12.0	14.2
Ala	11.8	7.8	13.4
Cys	2.4	1.4	n.d
Val	7.0	6.3	7.5
Met	0.5	3.2	3.1
Ile	5.3	7.2	10.9
Leu	11.1	11.5	15.5
Tyr	4.0	3.5	1.0
Phe	8.0	6.3	7.2

[a]Ref. 12.

[b]Ref. 21.

[c]Ref. 15.

particularly significant. A criterion often used to distinguish intrinsic membrane proteins from extrinsic and non-membrane proteins is that the intrinsic membrane proteins are not soluble in aqueous buffers. The solubility of membrane proteins clearly depends on the way they have been handled.

IV. DETERGENT SOLUBILIZATION OF MEMBRANE PROTEINS

Attempts to isolate and purify membrane proteins in a native form and in aqueous buffers have mostly employed detergents. These molecules, like phospholipids, are amphipathic structures with an apolar end of aliphatic or aromatic character and a polar end, which may be charged or uncharged [23]. Several common detergents are shown in Figure 2. Detergents differ from lipids in being more hydrophilic and therefore more water-soluble [24]. For example, sodium dodecyl sulfate (SDS) has a monomer solubility of about 10^{-2} M [25], whereas the solubility of monomers of dipalmitoyllecithin is 10^{-10} M [26]. The increased solubility of detergents over lipids derives from their ability to form micelles in aqueous solution.

Apparently, detergents are incorporated into the lipid bilayer of membranes as monomers [23, 27]. As their concentration in the membrane increases, they solubilize the membrane components by forming mixed micelles, some containing only lipid and detergent and others containing protein, lipid, and detergent [28, 29]. This process is shown schematically in Figure 3.

There is some indication that detergent monomers do not become intercalated into membranes randomly but are preferentially soluble in certain lipid or protein domains [30, 31]. Thus detergents can show a differential effect towards the proteins and lipids they solubilize, a fact used to advantage in enzyme purification. For example, deoxycholate solubilizes cytochromes b and c_1 from the mitochondrial inner membrane at concentrations of detergent much lower than those needed to release cytochrome c oxidase [30]. Lysolecithin can be used to solubilize the oligomycin-sensitive ATPase from this membrane at concentrations in which it leaves the cytochromes in a membranous pellet [32].

The binding of detergents to both membrane proteins and non-membrane proteins has been examined [for review, 23]. Based on their effect on protein conformation, detergents can be divided into denaturing and nondenaturing amphiphiles. Among the nondenaturing detergents, deoxycholate, cholate, and Triton X-100 are most commonly used in membrane studies. These detergents have been used to deplete membrane proteins of bound lipid [33–36]. When membrane fragments are incubated in the presence of a large excess of detergent, exchange of bound lipid with the detergent is favored and most proteins can be obtained in a lipid-free form, protein-detergent micelles being separated from lipid-detergent micelles by sucrose gradient centrifugation [37] or column chromatography [38].

Cytochrome c oxidase is one protein not freed of lipid by detergent exchange [39]. Several detergents have been tried and all exchange for the bulk of the lipid bound to the surface of this protein but leave attached several molecules of cardiolipin [39, 40]. These few molecules of cardiolipin can be dissociated from the enzyme only under conditions that denature the protein and dissociate it into its component polypeptides, that is, with strong organic solvents or in the presence of denaturing detergents such as SDS [39, 40].

The binding of detergents to several membrane proteins individually has been studied. Robinson and Tanford [41] have examined the association of both deoxycholate and Triton X-100 with the microsomal enzyme cytochrome b_5. Both detergents fail to bind to the enzyme when present at

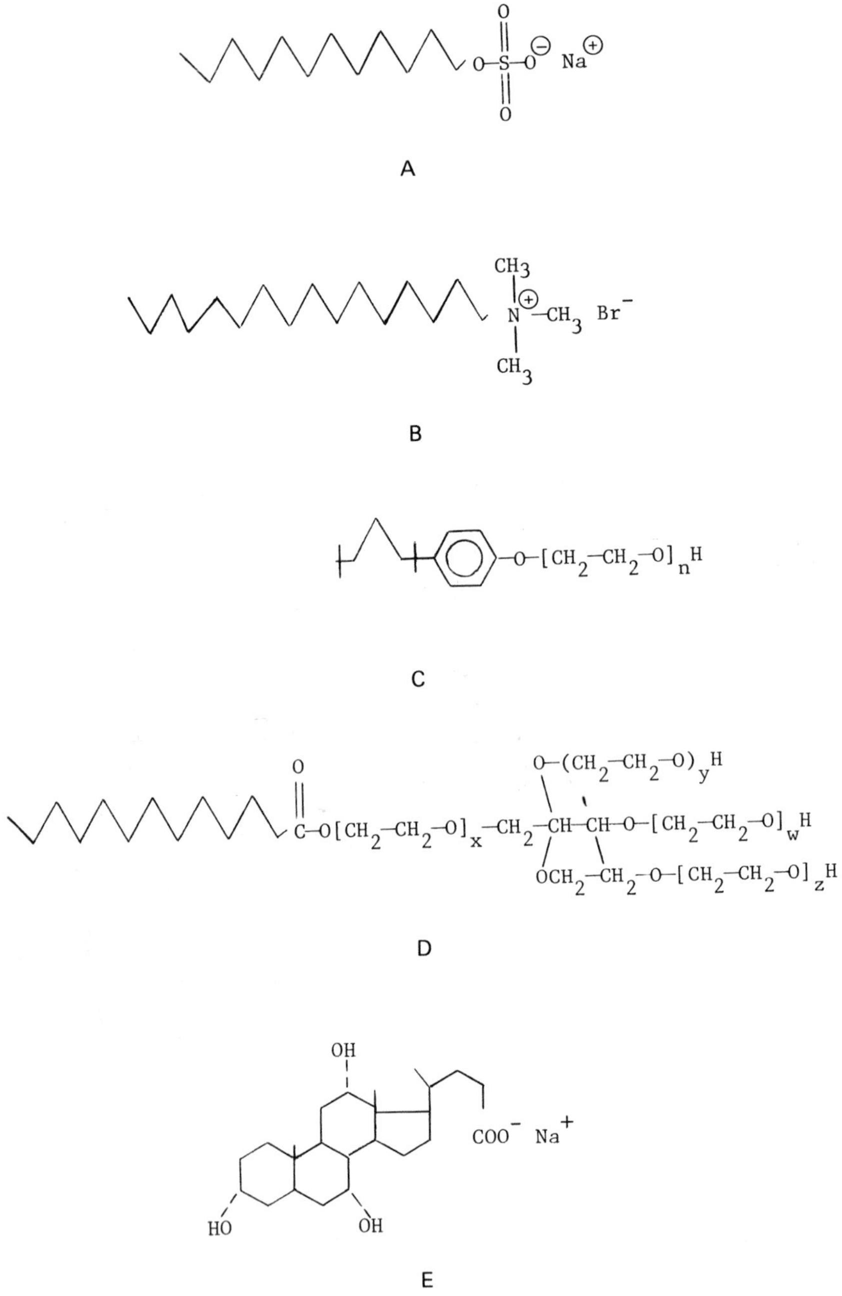

FIG. 2 Structure of several detergents commonly used in membrane studies. A. Sodium dodecyl sulfate. B. Cetyltrimethyl-ammonium bromide. C. Polyoxyethylene p-t-octyl phenols, e.g., Triton X series. D. Polyoxyethylene sorbitol esters, e.g., Tween series. E. Sodium cholate.

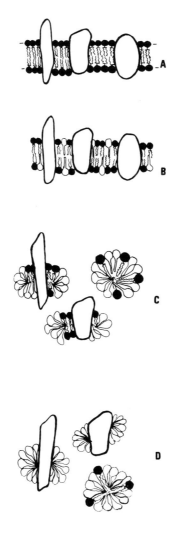

FIG. 3 A schematic representation of detergent solubilization of membranes. Detergents are thought to penetrate the membrane continuum (A, B)
in monomer form, until a concentration of detergent is reached (C) at which
protein-lipid-detergent mixed micelles are formed and the membrane is
thus solubilized. Additional detergent then separates proteins and lipids
into (D) protein–detergent mixed micelles and lipid–detergent mixed micelles.

TABLE 2

Binding of TX100 to Different Membrane Proteins

Protein	Detergent bound (mg/mg protein)	Reference
Cytochrome b_5	0.40	41
Rhodopsin	1.46	35
	1.10	47
Cholinergic receptor	0.30	42
ATPase SR	0.60	44
	0.20	47
Na^+-K^+ ATPase	0.28	47
Glycophorin	1.12	47
Cytochrome c oxidase	0.58	39
Cytochrome c	> 0.02	47
Glyceraldehyde-3-P-dehydrogenase	0.02	47

concentrations below their critical micelle concentration (c.m.c.). They bind in large amount, however, at concentrations above their c.m.c. Studies on the binding of nondenaturing detergents to several other membrane proteins show that the binding of these amphiphiles is a general property of intrinsic membrane proteins [28, 33, 35, 41-44]. These detergents most probably bind to the hydrophobic surface or surfaces of the protein that would in vivo interact with the fatty acid tails of lipid molecules [23, 41]. In contrast, nondenaturing detergents do not bind to either non-membrane proteins or

TABLE 3

Lipid-Free and Water-Soluble Complexes of Intrinsic Membrane Protein[a]

	Average No. Proteins	Reference
Neuraminidase spikes (Influenza virus)	12	48
Haemagglutinin spikes (Influenza virus)	5	48
Cytochrome b_5	8	34, 49
Cytochrome b_5 reductase	14	50
Cytochrome f.	8	51
Ca^{2+} ATPase SR	3.5	52
Semiliki Forest virus spikes	8	23

[a]Adapted from Ref. 23.

extrinsic proteins except in the rare case of protein whose physiological function is to bind amphiphiles, for example, serum albumins [45, 46].

The number of detergent molecules bound to several different membrane proteins has been measured. The number is large in all cases and is consistent with the formation of mixed micelles of protein and detergent (Table 2).

It is possible in some cases to remove bound detergents from membrane proteins and obtain a water-soluble preparation, but this depends on the manner in which the detergent is removed [23]. In all cases the soluble species is an aggregate that is presumably organized as a protein micelle with hydrophobic surfaces enclosed within the interior of the structure (Table 3).

V. BINDING OF DENATURING DETERGENTS AND USE IN SUBUNIT STRUCTURE ANALYSIS OF MEMBRANE PROTEINS

A wide range of denaturing detergents is available and two, sodium dodecyl sulfate and tetradecyltrimethyl-amoninium chloride, have been the most closely studied. These detergents bind to both membrane proteins and non-membrane proteins at concentrations below their c.m.c. [23]. SDS has been used extensively as the detergent for polyacrylamide-gel electrophoretic examination of the subunit structure of membrane (and non-membrane) protein.

Sodium dodecyl sulfate is the detergent of choice in these studies because of its observed binding properties and structural effects on non-membrane proteins. It is a strong denaturant, and proteins are usually dissociated into their constituent polypeptide chains by its action [53-55]. Also, the reduced polypeptide chains form detergent protein complexes in which the protein is saturated with about 1.4 g of SDS per g of protein [56, 57]. This large amount of bound anionic detergent swamps out any effect the net charge of the protein might have on its migration in gels. Finally the SDS-polypeptide complex forms an extended rodlike particle having a length roughly proportional to the molecular weight of the polypeptides [58]. The molecular weights of proteins which behave as just described can be obtained by comparing their migration with the migration of standard proteins of known molecular weight run on companion gels [53, 54]. Unfortunately, many membrane proteins behave anomalously. Hydrophobic polypeptides appear to bind more than 1.4 g SDS per g protein [59, 60]. Grefath and Reynolds [59] find that the MN glycoprotein of the red-cell membrane binds more than 5 g SDS per g of protein. Also, membrane proteins, again particularly the hydrophobic ones, can have an intrinsic stability towards unfolding in SDS [61] and their migration then depends on the conditions used to dissociate the complex. Only after being heated in SDS, or when

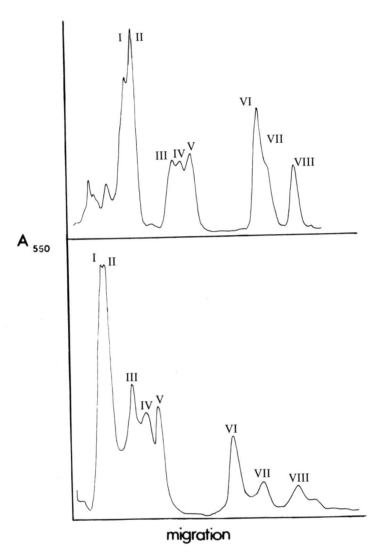

FIG. 4 Densitometric traces of ubiquinone cytochrome c reductase run on 12% polyacrylamide gels in a buffer system containing SDS alone (top gel) and SDS plus 8 M urea (bottom gel). Bands are labeled I-VIII. Reproduced from [68], with the kind permission of the American Chemical Society.

8 M urea is included along with SDS in the dissociating buffer, are these polypeptides fully unfolded.

The stability of certain proteins in SDS can be used to advantage in enzyme purification. A b-type cytochrome of the complex III segment of the mitochrondrial respiratory chain has been purified by dissociating this complex in 1% SDS at room temperature, conditions that dissociate and denature other polypeptides of the complex but leave the b heme-bearing component untouched [62].

It has proven difficult to ascertain how many different polypeptides there are in several membrane protein complexes. It is possible that any band in gels contains two or more polypeptides that happen to comigrate under the conditions in which the gels are being run. One approach to ruling this out is to use two-dimensional electrophoresis, in which components are separated in one dimension by isoelectric focusing and in a second dimension by electrophoresis in SDS [63]. It has been shown that proteins dissociated and denatured by SDS can be subjected to isoelectric focusing in 8 M urea when high levels of Triton X-100 or other non-ionic detergent are added [63, 64]. During electrophoresis, the SDS is replaced on the surface of proteins by non-ionic detergent and the former detergent is electrophoresed out of the gels as an SDS/non-ionic detergent mixed micelle. After isoelectric focusing, SDS is introduced into the gel and the polypeptides are electrophoresed into a slab gel, through which they migrate in proportion to their size [63, 65].

Proteins or protein complexes that contain low-molecular-weight polypeptides are particularly difficult to resolve completely by the usual gel methods. Components with molecular weights of 10,000 and lower migrate close together along with SDS micelles [58, 66]. They can be separated, however, if 8 M urea is included in gels along with SDS [67]. The improved resolution with 8 M urea is clear from our studies with ubiquinone-cytochrome c reductase [68]. This complex is resolved into several high-molecular-weight polypeptides and three closely spaced bands with molecular weights between 16,000 and 9000 when electrophoresed in SDS alone. In SDS and 8 M urea, these fast-migrating bands become widely separated and run with molecular weights of from 12,000 to 4400 (Fig. 4).

VI. PRIMARY STRUCTURE OF MEMBRANE PROTEINS

Intrinsic membrane proteins are by definition partly buried in a hydrocarbon environment and must present an apolar face to the lipids. Those most deeply buried in the bilayer have much of their surface in contact with lipid and they can be expected, compared with non-membrane proteins, to contain an increased number of hydrophobic amino acids. Early attempts to confirm this were inconclusive since workers were comparing the amino acid composition of whole membranes (including both intrinsic and extrinsic proteins) with amino acids of water-soluble non-membrane proteins [69, 70]. The first attempt to analyze purified membrane proteins compared the sum of

TABLE 4

Polarities of Some Intrinsic Membrane Proteins

A. Single polypeptide chains of overall low polarity

Protein	Polarity (%)	Reference
Folch-Lees proteolipid from sciatic myelin	29	12
C_{55} isoprenoid alcohol phosphokinase	31	81
Purple membrane protein Halobacterium halobium	34	84
Rhodopsin, bovine	36	80, 82
Carotenoid glycoprotein Sarcina Flava	38	83
ATPase stearylcoenzyme A desaturase	38	79

B. Single polypeptide chains, a fragment of which has a low overall polarity

Protein	Polarity of hydro-phobic fragments (%)	Reference
Cytochrome b_5	30	34
Cytochrome b_5 reductase	35	85
Semiliki Forest virus glycoproteins	28	86
Sucrose isomaltase from the pig small intestine	30	87
Aminopeptidase from the intestine brush border	35	88

C. Multipeptide aggregates or complexes, component peptides of which have a low polarity

Proteins	Subunits by MW	Polarity (%)	Reference
Reaction centers from Rhodopseudomonas spheroides	21,000	29	
	24,000	30	89
	28,000	38	
Cytochrome c oxidase, beef heart	35,400	36	72, 73
	24,100	45	
	21,000	40	
	16,800	49	
	12,400	48	
	8,200	50	
	4,400	45	

the mole percentage of Lys, His, Arg, Asp, Ser, Thr, and Glu, the so-called polarity of these proteins, with the polarity of a large number of non-membrane proteins [71]. It was found that 85% of the 205 soluble proteins considered had polarities of 47±6% and only 2% had polarities below 40%. Almost half the membrane proteins examined at that time had polarities below 40%. Most of these were proteins deeply buried in the lipid bilayer [71] (Table 4).

For many membrane proteins, only a small portion of the protein appears to be buried within the bilayer. In these, a fragment of the protein might be expected to have a low polarity. This appears to be the case and a segment of individual polypeptides or one or more subunits of multimeric enzymes has been found to contain a concentration of hydrophobic amino acids [68, 72, 73, 74] [Table 4].

Several membrane proteins, including the MN glycoprotein [75], a lipoprotein of $\underline{E}$. $\underline{coli}$ [76], and a coat protein of coliphage M13 [77], have been sequenced. Both the MN glycoprotein and the coat protein have extended sequences of hydrophobic amino acids, as discussed in this book by Segrest and Jackson. This had led Segrest and Feldmann [78] to look for long sequences of hydrophobic amino acids in proteins that are both membrane and non-membrane in origin, with the idea that this might prove a feature unique to membrane proteins and of structural importance to them. A sequence rich in hydrophobic amino acids is not a feature of $\underline{E}$. $\underline{coli}$ lipoprotein [76].

VII. SECONDARY STRUCTURE OF MEMBRANE PROTEINS

Non-membrane proteins show a diversity of structures from predominantly random coil to a fully alpha-helical conformation. An alpha-helical structure provides a stable arrangement of protein in a hydrocarbon environment [90], and consequently it has been suggested that this is the preferred conformation of intrinsic membrane proteins [3, 91]. An alpha-helical structure of these proteins has also been inferred from model-building studies. Predictions of conformation made on the basis of known amino acid sequences have fairly successfully identified regions of alpha helix in several non-membrane proteins, judged by reference to their X-ray structure [92-96]. These formulations have been applied to the few intrinsic membrane proteins of known sequences and each has the characteristics of a highly alpha-helical polypeptide [97].

Attempts to show an alpha-helical structure of membrane proteins experimentally have mostly used circular dichroism (CD) or optical rotatory dispersion (ORD) studies of whole membrane preparations [91, 98, for reviews]. Interpreting the spectra obtained in these experiments has proved difficult because the bands are shifted in comparison with those seen in non-membrane proteins. The CD spectra of model alpha-helical polypeptides contain negative bands at 222 nm and 208 nm and a positive band at 192 nm. The CD spectra of biological membranes, however, show all extrema at longer wavelengths, with the magnitude of the bands near 208 and 192 nm markedly reduced relative to bands near 222 nm [98]. These spectral shifts and damping effects have been attributed to light-scattering artifacts due to the particulate nature of the samples [91, 98].

Clear evidence for the predominantly alpha-helical arrangement of at least one membrane protein has been obtained in the recent work of Henderson and Unwin [99, 100] on the purple membrane protein of Halobacterium halobium. These workers have used the electron microscope to get an electron diffraction map of the purple membrane to 7 Å, a level of resolution that shows the conformation of the peptide backbone as a series of alpha helixes amounting to 70%-80% of the protein structure [100].

Evidence for beta structure in membrane proteins has been obtained by several laboratories using infrared spectroscopy. The amide I band in IR spectra of proteins is due primarily to $C=O$ stretching of the polypeptide backbone. This band is conformationally sensitive, its intensity and spectral position varying with hydrogen bonding at the $C=O$. For alpha helical or random coil structure, the band maximum is around $1,650$ cm^{-1}, but for beta structure the maximum shifts to $1,635$ cm^{-1} and there is a shoulder at $1,685$ cm^{-1} [101 for review]. Infrared spectra of Micrococcus lysodekticus membrane [102], Acholeplasma laidlawii membrane [103], adiposite plasma membranes [104], and mitochondrial membranes [105] all show evidence of beta structure.

Among other approaches to examining the conformation of membrane proteins, the hydrogen-exchange technique appears to hold considerable promise. Downer and Englander [106] have used this method to examine the structure of rhodopsin in the retinal rod membrane. Their results indicate that this protein is relatively unstructured although X-ray diffraction data suggest that the polypeptide is fairly deeply buried in the lipid bilayer. The same method applied to purple membrane protein shows a large amount of structured polypeptide, as expected if this protein is in predominantly alpha-helical arrangement [107].

VIII. ON THE DISTINCTION BETWEEN INTRINSIC AND EXTRINSIC
       MEMBRANE PROTEINS

Before 1972, the generally accepted picture of biomembranes was an uninterrupted lipid bilayer with protein distributed exclusively on the surface of the continuum. With the recent acceptance of the notion that protein can be an integral part of the membrane continuum, a big question in membrane research is how to develop ways of distinguishing between these intrinsic membrane proteins and extrinsic, or peripheral, membrane proteins. Is there more than a descriptional difference between these classes of proteins?

There have been several attempts to define properties that will distinguish intrinsic membrane proteins from extrinsic and non-membrane proteins. Singer [108], for example, has proposed three distinguishing criteria
as follows.

1. Extrinsic membrane proteins are released from membranes under
   mild conditions that do not disrupt the lipid bilayer, such as changes
   in salt concentration and the presence of metal chelating agents.
   Intrinsic membrane proteins on the other hand require hydrophobic
   bond-breaking agents to release them from their respective membranes.
2. Extrinsic membrane proteins are released from a membrane free
   of lipid whereas intrinsic proteins have associated lipid as solubilized.
3. Extrinsic membrane proteins are soluble and molecularly dispersed
   in neutral aqueous buffers, whereas intrinsic proteins as released
   from membranes are aggregated in neutral aqueous buffers.

The first criterion is of experimental use in examining individual membranes but by no means all-inclusive in deciding which proteins are extrinsic
or intrinsic to a particular membrane. Many different proteins can be
released from membrane by mild conditions. Thus spectrin, glyceraldehyde
3-dehydrogenase, a Ca^{2+} ATPase, and in all up to 50% of the membrane-
associated protein, can be solubilized from red-cell ghosts by low salt,
or with low concentration of EDTA [for review, 109]. Cytochrome c
among other polypeptides can be removed from the mitochondrial inner
membrane by low salt treatment [110]. These components can all be identified as extrinsic, or peripheral, to the lipid bilayer. Unfortunately, not all
extrinsic membrane proteins are necessarily removed by mild conditions.
Proteins localized exclusively on the outside of the lipid bilayer can make
hydrophobic contacts with proteins that are themselves intrinsic to the
membrane continuum, and these would require hydrophobic bond-breaking
conditions to be released. The mitochondrial ATPase [111], cytochrome c_1
[112], and calsequestin (from the sarcoplasmic reticulum) [113] are among
the extrinsic membrane proteins that require chaotropic salts or detergents
to release them from their respective membranes.

Other criteria, such as solubility in neutral aqueous buffer and presence
of lipid as solubilized, do not provide an experimental basis for distinguishing the two classes. As discussed earlier, many intrinsic membrane proteins have been obtained in a water-soluble and lipid-free form and the final
state of these proteins depends on the conditions used for their isolation.
The key structural difference between intrinsic membrane proteins and
extrinsic proteins or non-membrane proteins appears to be in the properties
of their surfaces. Intrinsic membrane proteins must provide a hydrophobic
surface for a stable interaction with lipids. In extreme cases this results
in an increased hydrophobic character, or to use one measure of this, they

have a low polarity. Alternatively, there may be very hydrophobic segments of polypeptide chain in these proteins. The presence of hydrophobic pockets on the surface of intrinsic proteins results in their binding nondenaturing detergents. Extrinsic proteins and non-membrane proteins with a few exceptions do not bind these detergents, and (as first suggested by Helenius and Simons [23]; see also Chapter 6) detergent binding may be one experimental method by which to decide which proteins in any membrane are intrinsic to the lipid bilayer.

REFERENCES

1. R. A. Capaldi and D. E. Green, FEBS Letters, 25, 205 (1972).
2. G. Vanderkooi, Ann. N.Y. Acad. Sci., 195, 6 (1972).
3. S. J. Singer and G. L. Nicolson, Science, 175, 720 (1972).
4. O. O. Blumenfeld, P. M. Gallop, C. Howe, and L. T. Lee, Biochim. Biophys. Acta, 211, 109 (1970).
5. V. T. Marchesi and E. P. Andrews, Science, 174, 1247 (1971).
6. H. Hamaguchi and H. Cleve, Biochim. Biophys. Acta, 278, 271 (1972).
7. R. J. Winzler, in Red Cell Membrane Structure and Function, ed. G. A. Jamieson and T. Z. Greenwalt. Philadelphia: J. B. Lippincott, 1969, p. 157.
8. A. H. Maddy, Biochim. Biophys. Acta, 117, 193 (1966).
9. H. P. Zahler and D. F. H. Wallach, Biochim. Biophys. Acta, 135, 371 (1967).
10. J. Folch-Pi and P. J. Stoffyn, Ann. N.Y. Acad. Sci., 195, 86 (1972).
11. J. Folch and M. Lees, J. Biol. Chem., 191, 807 (1951).
12. L. R. Eng, F. C. Chao, B. Gerstl, D. Pratt, and M. G. Tavaststyema, Biochemistry, 7, 4455 (1968).
13. M. J. Rowe, R. A. Lansman, and D. O. Woodward, Eur. J. Biochemistry, 41, 25 (1974).
14. B. Kadenbach and P. Hadvary, Eur. J. Biochemistry, 32, 343 (1973).
15. M. F. Sierra and A. Tzagoloff, Proc. Nat. Acad. Sci. U.S., 70, 3155 (1973).
16. D. H. MacLennan, C. C. Yip, G. H. Iles, and P. Seaman, Cold Spring Harbor Symposium Quant. Biology, 37, 469 (1972).
17. S. F. Plasas and E. De Robertis, Biochim. Biophys. Acta, 224, 258 (1972).
18. M. Parisi, T. A. Reader, and E. De Robertis, J. Gen. Physiol., 60, 454 (1972).
19. T. A. Reader, M. Parisi, and E. De Robertis, Biochem. Biophys. Res. Commun., 53, 10 (1973).
20. G. Schatz and T. Mason, Ann. Rev. Biochem., 43, 51 (1974).
21. R. O. Poyton and G. Schatz, J. Biol. Chem., 250, 752 (1975).
22. D. Tennenbaum and J. Folch-Pi, Biochim. Biophys. Acta, 115, 141 (1963).

23. A. Helenius and K. Simons, Biochim. Biophys. Acta, 415, 29 (1975).
24. D. M. Small, Fed. Proc., 29, 1320 (1970).
25. P. Mukerjee and K. J. Mysels, Critical Micelle Concentrations in Aqueous Surfactant Systems. Washington: National Bureau of Standards NSRDS-NBS 36, 1971.
26. C. Tanford, J. Mol. Biol., 67, 59 (1972).
27. R. Smith and C. Tanford, J. Mol. Biol., 67, 75 (1972).
28. K. Simons, A. Helenius, and H. Garoff, J. Mol. Biol., 80, 119 (1973).
29. A. Helenius and H. Soderlund, Biochim. Biophys. Acta, 307, 287 (1973).
30. F. L. Crane and J. D. Hall, Ann. N.Y. Acad. Sci., 195, 24 (1972).
31. F. H. Kirkpatrick, S. E. Gordesky, and G. V. Marinetti, Biochim. Biophys. Acta, 345, 154 (1974).
32. M. H. Sadler, D. R. Hunter, and R. A. Haworth, Biochem. Biophys. Res. Commun., 59, 804 (1974).
33. A. Helenius and K. Simons, J. Biol. Chem., 247, 3656 (1972).
34. L. Spatz and P. Strittmatter, Proc. Nat. Acad. Sci. U.S., 68, 1042 (1971).
35. B. H. Osborn, G. Sardet, and A. Helenius, Eur. J. Biochem., 44, 383 (1974).
36. D. Allan and M. J. Crumpton, Biochem. J., 123, 967 (1971).
37. D. M. Engelman, T. M. Terry, and H. J. Morowitz, Biochim. Biophys. Acta, 135, 381 (1967).
38. E. E. Jacobs, F. H. Kirkpatrick, B. C. Andrews, W. Cunningham, and F. L. Crane, Biochem. Biophys. Res. Commun., 25, 96 (1966).
39. N. C. Robinson and R. A. Capaldi, Biochemistry, 16, 375 (1977).
40. Y. C. Awasthi, T. F. Chuang, T. W. Keenan, and F. L. Crane, Biochim. Biophys. Acta, 226, 42 (1971).
41. N. C. Robinson and C. Tanford, Biochemistry, 14, 369 (1975).
42. J. C. Meunier, R. W. Olsen, and J. P. Changeaux, FEBS Letters, 24, 63 (1972).
43. M. S. Rubin and A. Tzagoloff, J. Biol. Chem., 248, 4269 (1973).
44. H. Walter and W. Hasselbach, Eur. J. Biochem., 44, 383 (1973).
45. S. Makino, J. A. Reynolds, and C. Tanford, J. Biol. Chem., 248, 4926 (1973).
46. P. A. Albertsson, Biochemistry, 12, 2525 (1973).
47. S. Clarke, J. Biol. Chem., 250, 5459 (1975).
48. W. G. Laver and R. C. Valentine, Virology, 38, 105 (1969).
49. A. Ito and R. Sato, J. Biol. Chem., 243, 4922 (1968).
50. L. Spatz and P. Strittmatter, J. Mol. Biol., 248, 793 (1973).
51. N. Nelson and E. Racker, J. Biol. Chem., 247, 3848 (1972).
52. P. M. D. Hardwicke and N. M. Green, Eur. J. Biochem., 42, 183 (1974).
53. A. L. Shapiro, E. Vinuela, and J. V. Maizel, Biochem. Biophys. Res. Commun., 28, 815 (1967).
54. K. Weber and M. Osborn, J. Biol. Chem., 244, 4406 (1969).

55. W. W. Fish, J. A. Reynolds, and C. Tanford, J. Biol. Chem., 245, 5166 (1970).
56. R. Pitt-Rivers and F. S. A. Impiombato, Biochem. J., 109, 825 (1968).
57. J. A. Reynolds and C. Tanford, Proc. Nat. Acad. Sci. U.S., 66, 1002 (1970).
58. J. A. Reynolds and C. Tanford, J. Biol. Chem., 245, 5161 (1970).
59. S. P. Grefath and J. A. Reynolds, Proc. Nat. Acad. Sci. U.S., 71, 3913 (1974).
60. N. C. Robinson and R. A. Capaldi, unpublished studies.
61. R. L. Bell and R. A. Capaldi, unpublished studies.
62. C. A. Yu, L. Yu, and T. E. King, Biochem. Biophys. Res. Commun., 66, 1194 (1975).
63. P. H. O'Farrel, J. Biol. Chem., 250, 4007 (1975).
64. R. Ruchel, S. Mesecke, D. Wolfourn, and V. Neuhoff, Hoppe Seylers Z. Physiol. Chem., 355, 997 (1974).
65. G. F.-L. Ames and N. Nikaido, Biochemistry, 15, 616 (1976).
66. J. B. Williams and W. B. Gratzer, J. Chromatogr., 57, 121 (1971).
67. R. T. Swank and K. D. Munkres, Anal. Biochem., 39, 462 (1971).
68. R. L. Bell and R. A. Capaldi, Biochemistry, 15, 996 (1976).
69. F. T. Hatch and A. L. Bruce, Nature, 218, 1166 (1968).
70. D. F. H. Wallach and A. Gordon, Nature Fed. Proc., 27, 1263 (1968).
71. R. A. Capaldi and G. Vanderkooi, Proc. Nat. Acad. Sci. U.S., 69, 930 (1972).
72. M. Briggs, P. F. Kamp, N. C. Robinson, and R. A. Capaldi, Biochemistry, 14, 5123 (1975).
73. N. W. Downer, N. C. Robinson, and R. A. Capaldi, Biochemistry, 15, 2930 (1976).
74. R. O. Poyton and G. Schatz, J. Biol. Chem., 250, 752 (1975).
75. M. Tomita and V. T. Marchesi, Proc. Nat. Acad. Sci. U.S., 72, 2964 (1975).
76. V. Braun, Biochim. Biophys. Acta, 415, 335 (1975).
77. Y. Nakashuna, R. L. Wiseman, W. Konigsber, and D. A. Marvin, Nature, 253, 68 (1975).
78. J. P. Segrest and R. J. Feldmann, J. Mol. Biol., 87, 853 (1974).
79. P. Strittmatter, L. Spatz, D. Corcoran, M. J. Rogers, B. Setlow, and R. Redline, Proc. Nat. Acad. Sci. U.S., 71, 4565 (1974).
80. W. E. Robinson, A. Gordon-Walker, and D. Bownds, Nature, 235, 112 (1972).
81. H. Sandermann and J. L. Strominger, Proc. Nat. Acad. Sci. U.S., 68, 2441 (1971).
82. J. Heller, Biochemistry, 7, 2906 (1968).
83. D. Thurkell and M. I. S. Hunter, J. Gen. Microbiol., 58, 289 (1969).
84. W. Stoeckenius and W. H. Kanau, J. Cell Biol., 38, 337 (1968).
85. L. Spatz and P. Strittmatter, J. Biol. Chem., 248, 793 (1972).
86. G. Utermann and K. Simons, J. Mol. Biol., 85, 569 (1974).

87. H. Sigrist, P. Ronner, and G. Semenza, Biochim. Biophys. Acta, 406, 433 (1975).
88. S. Maroux and P. Louvard, Biochim. Biophys. Acta, 419, 189 (1976).
89. L. A. Steiner, M. Y. Okamura, A. D. Lopes, E. Moskowitz, and G. Feher, Biochemistry, 13, 1403 (1974).
90. G. D. Fasman, in Poly-α-amino Acids, ed. G. D. Fasman. London: Edward Arnold, 1967, p. 499.
91. D. F. H. Wallach and R. J. Winzler, Evolving Strategies and Tactics in Membrane Research. New York, Heidelberg, Berlin: Springer Verlag, 1974.
92. G. E. Schultz, C. D. Barry, J. Friedman, P. Y. Chou, G. D. Fasman, A. V. Finkelstein, V. I. Lim, O. B. Ptitsyn, E. A. Kabat, T. T. Wu, M. Levitt, B. Robson, and K. Nagano, Nature, 250, 140 (1974).
93. P. Y. Chou and G. D. Fasman, Biochemistry, 13, 211 (1974).
94. P. Y. Chou and G. D. Fasman, Biochemistry, 13, 222 (1974).
95. V. I. Lim, J. Mol. Biol., 88, 857 (1974).
96. V. I. Lim, J. Mol. Biol., 88, 873 (1974).
97. N. M. Green and M. T. Flanagan, Biochem. J., 153, 729 (1976).
98. D. Urry, Biochim. Biophys. Acta, 265, 115 (1972).
99. N. Unwin and R. Henderson, J. Mol. Biol., 94, 425 (1975).
100. R. Henderson and N. Unwin, Nature, 257, 28 (1975).
101. D. F. H. Wallach and R. J. Winzler, Evolving Strategies and Tactics in Membrane Research. New York, Heidelberg, Berlin: Springer Verlag, 1974, p. 140.
102. D. H. Green and M. R. J. Salton, Biochim. Biophys. Acta, 211, 139 (1970).
103. G. L. Choules and R. F. Bjorklund, Biochemistry, 9, 4759 (1970).
104. J. Avruch and D. F. H. Wallach, Biochim. Biophys. Acta, 241, 249 (1971).
105. D. F. H. Wallach, J. M. Graham, and B. R. Ferbach, Arch. Biochem. Biophys., 131, 322 (1969).
106. N. Downer and W. Englander, Nature, 254, 625 (1975).
107. N. Downer, personal communication.
108. S. J. Singer, Ann. Rev. Biochem., 43, 805 (1974).
109. T. L. Steck, J. Cell Biol., 62, 1 (1974).
110. E. E. Jacobs and D. R. Sanadi, J. Biol. Chem., 235, 531 (1960).
111. M. E. Pullman, H. S. Penefsky, A. Datta, and E. Racker, J. Biol. Chem., 235, 3322 (1960).
112. Y. Orii and K. Okunuki, Ann. Rept. Biol. Works Faculty Sci. Osaka Univ., 17, 1 (1969).
113. D. H. MacLennan and P. T. S. Wong, Proc. Nat. Acad. Sci. U.S., 68, 1231 (1971).

Chapter 2

MOLECULAR PROPERTIES OF MEMBRANE PROTEINS
A Comparison of Transverse and Surface Lipid Association Sites

Jere P. Segrest

Comprehensive Cancer Center
Department of Pathology
Birmingham Medical Center
Birmingham, Alabama

Richard L. Jackson

Department of Medicine
Baylor College of Medicine
and
The Methodist Hospital
Houston, Texas

I. INTRODUCTION

The nature of the interactions between the protein and lipid constituents of
cellular membranes and of other lipid-protein complexes, such as the plasma
lipoproteins, is of considerable immediate interest. Part of this is a result
of recent evidence that the regulation of cell growth and division is membrane-
mediated [1] and that defects in membrane function may relate to cancer [2].
In addition, there is considerable evidence that the plasma lipoproteins are
very important in the pathophysiology of atherosclerosis [3].

    Biological membranes in the abstract may be considered sheets of
aqueous discontinuity. It is generally accepted that a phospholipid bilayer
provides the basic structural and functional skeleton for membranes [4-8].
It is clear, however, that lipids alone do not mediate the wide variety of
complex biological functions performed by the membranes of cells. Since
these functions are undoubtedly mediated by membrane proteins, understanding the mechanisms for controlling such cell surface phenomena as ion
and metabolite transport, and receptor and surface antigen-mediated transmembrane signals, requires a knowledge of the topomolecular organization
of proteins relative to the basic lipid organizational unit, the bilayer. Similarly, knowing how the protein components of plasma lipoproteins are organized relative to the lipids is necessary in order to understand the details of
the transport and metabolism of lipids.

II. PROTEINS WITH HIGH LIPID AFFINITY

A. Cytochrome b_5

Because of recent advances in methodology for isolating membrane constituents, numerous proteins with high lipid affinities are now being studied. One
such protein is cytochrome b_5, which is a component of the liver microsomal
membrane. It has been shown that this protein is composed of two distinct
domains [9], one hydrophobic and the second hydrophilic. The NH_2-terminal,
or hydrophilic, domain of the protein has a molecular weight of 11,000 and
can be released from microsomes by treating the membranes with trypsin
[10]. The amino acid sequence and three-dimensional structure of this
domain have been determined; the domain has the properties of a typical

globular protein [10]. The domain that remains in the membrane following trypsin treatment has a molecular weight of 5,000 and is rich in hydrophobic amino acids; the amino acid sequence of this domain has not been determined [9]. It has been shown, however, that this hydrophobic domain is required for incorporating the protein into either membranes or phosphatidylcholine vesicles [11]. From these findings, it is assumed that the hydrophobic domain of cytochrome b_5 at least partially penetrates the lipophilic interior of the microsomal membrane.

B. Rhodopsin

A second membrane protein whose manner of association with biological membranes has been studied is the light-sensitive protein rhodopsin. The protein from the membranes of frog retinal disc has a molecular weight of 40,000 [12]. Rhodopsin has been incorporated into phospholipid vesicles and has been demonstrated, by freeze-fracture electron microscopy, to form intramembranous particles of approximately 100Å in diameter [13, 14]. Recent X-ray diffraction studies have shown that rhodopsin is located on one side of the retinal disc membrane and penetrates the membrane approximately halfway [15]. No data are available on the relation of the primary and tertiary structures of rhodopsin to its association with membrane lipids.

C. Component A

A principal protein of the human red-cell membrane, designated component A by Bretscher [16] and protein III by Fairbanks et al. [17], has been shown by labeling and differential protease cleavage techniques to span the red-cell membrane [16, 18]. The protein appears to have a monomeric molecular weight of approximately 100,000 and forms multimeric units of either dimers [19] or tetramers [20]. Although the physiological function of this protein is not completely known, there is some evidence that protein III forms a chloride channel through the red-cell membrane [21, 22]. Protein III has recently been isolated and partially purified [22], but little is known about the primary and tertiary structures of protein III or its relation to the membrane bilayer. It is known, however, that the protein is associated with the intramembranous particles seen in the red-cell membrane [23].

D. Semliki Forest Virus Spike Glycoprotein

Semliki Forest virus spike glycoprotein is another membrane-spanning protein. This glycoprotein with a molecular weight of 50,000 appears to have a hydrophobic segment of approximately 50 amino acids that interacts with the hydrophobic core of the membrane [24]. The model suggested for the topomolecular anatomy of the Semliki Forest glycoprotein is similar to the

model for the MN-glycoprotein (glycophorin) of the red-cell membrane, to
be discussed below.

E. Filamentous Virus Coat Protein

The B coat protein from the filamentous bacteriophages (FV) is a membrane-
associating protein whose amino acid sequence has been known for some
time [25, 26]. This protein has not been generally recognized as a membrane
protein, however. We recently suggested [27, 51] on the basis of a computer
search for hydrophobic domains within proteins of known sequence that the
B phage protein was most likely a membrane protein. This is consistent with
observations that the coat protein is stored in the bacterial membrane during
replication of the phage within the bacteria [28] and associates strongly with
the lipids of the bacterial membrane [29]. The amino acid sequence of the
B coat protein contains three domains forming an amphipathic sandwich in
which the NH_2-terminal and COOH-terminal portions of the proteins are
highly charged and the intervening 19-residue segment is extremely hydrophobic [25, 76]. It seems probable that this protein when stored in the
bacterial membrane spans the membrane in a fashion similar to that suggested for the MN-glycoprotein of the red-cell membrane [30, 31] and the
Semliki Forest virus glycoprotein [24].

F. Gramicidin A

The polypeptide antibiotic gramicidin A is one of the first lipid-associated
"proteins" (polypeptides) to have had its molecular structure examined in
detail. This antibiotic consists of a polypeptide of 15 residues with alternating
L and D hydrophobic amino acid residues [32]. A specific molecular model
has been proposed by Urry [33] (recently modified by Veatch et al. [34]) for
the association of gramicidin A with biological membranes and artificial
lipid membranes. Urry proposes that gramicidin A forms a helical structure,
termed a $\beta^6 3,3$-helix, in the hydrocarbon core of the membrane bilayer
[33]. By virtue of a large number of residues per turn, the helical structure
would have a hollow center. Urry suggests that by means of head-to-head
dimerization, gramicidin A forms a channel across the bilayer for specific
cations [33]; cations are coordinated through the hollow center of the helix
and across the membrane. The dimer forms an extremely hydrophobic
membrane-spanning helix that is approximately 30Å long, the thickness of
the hydrophobic domain of a phospholipid bilayer [23].

G. Valinomycin and Alamethicin

Two bacterially derived lipid-associating polypeptides in addition to gramicidin A have been examined at the molecular level. Valinomycin is a cyclic

polypeptide ion carrier, which, it is postulated, forms hydrophobic rings around ions, allowing their diffusion across membranes [35]. Alamethicin, also a cyclic polypeptide, interacts in a coordinated fashion with itself, apparently to form multimeric channels across membranes that are hydrophobic on the outside and hydrophilic on the inside [36]. The geometrical properties of these channels have some similarities to the properties of the model to be discussed below for the hydrophobic domain of the human erythrocyte MN-glycoprotein.

Unfortunately, the polypeptides gramicidin A, valinomycin, and alamethicin, in addition to being bacterially derived and presumably not native components of the bacterial membrane, have singular properties such as unusual amino acid residues and cyclic structures; these seriously limit their usefulness as analogs for predicting properties of protein-lipid interactions associated with mammalian membranes and lipoproteins. Therefore, we should like to consider now in some detail the molecular properties of two mammalian lipid-associating polypeptide structures, one derived from an intrinsic membrane protein and the second from certain plasma apolipoproteins. Our thesis is that the molecular models derived for these two classes of lipid-associating proteins allow the derivation of certain generalities useful for predicting the properties of the lipid-associating domains of other apoproteins from mammalian membranes and lipoproteins.

III. MN-GLYCOPROTEIN

A glycoprotein containing the MN blood group activity was isolated by Winzler [37] and Morawiecki [38] from the human red-cell membrane over ten years ago. Independently, both authors proposed that this glycoprotein is anchored in the membrane by a hydrophobic segment at the COOH-terminal end of the molecule. This topomolecular model for the MN-glycoprotein (glycophorin) and its mode of association within the red-cell membrane has been modified by recent work of Marchesi and coworkers [30, 39, 40].

The MN-glycoprotein composes approximately 10 percent of the human erythrocyte membrane protein. The glycoprotein has receptor sites for phytohemagglutinin, influenza virus, and wheat germ agglutinin and carries the MN blood group antigens [40]. These receptors and antigens are contained in the NH_2-terminal portion of the glycoprotein and are exposed to the external milieu of the red cell [30, 40]. Initial chemical and structural characterizations of the MN-glycoprotein have shown that it has a molecular weight of approximately 31,000 [41, 42] and contains a carbohydrate-rich NH_2-terminal region, a hydrophilic COOH terminus rich in proline residues but containing no carbohydrate, and an intervening nonpolar domain [30, 39, 40]. Labeling studies, using lactoperoxidase-catalyzed iodination of the glycoprotein tyrosine residues in situ on erythrocytes and erythrocyte ghosts of varying degrees of permeability, suggest that the NH_2 terminus and COOH terminus of the glycoprotein are on opposite sides of the membrane; viz., the NH_2 terminus is extracellular (as the plant lectin and MN blood group sites are) and the COOH terminus intracellular [30].

The MN-glycoprotein is also associated with intramembranous particles located in the hydrophobic core of the erythrocyte membrane. Tillack et al. [43] used phytohemagglutinin (PHA) conjugated with ferritin to produce complexes that were able to be discerned by freeze-etch electron microscopy; PHA binds to the MN-glycoprotein sites on the surface of erythrocyte membranes. By a combination of fracture and etching, these workers demonstrated that MN-glycoprotein is associated with the particles. The MN-glycoprotein corresponded exactly to the distribution of intramembranous particles, even when the distribution of the latter was markedly altered [43].

Since the MN-glycoprotein spans the membrane, the amino acid sequence of those residues associated with the phospholipid bilayer is of interest. This portion of the molecule is hydrophobic and is contained intact within a hydrophobic tryptic peptide T(is) (35 residues and a residue weight of 3,700) produced from MN-glycoprotein. The amino acid sequence [39] of this peptide (plus 5 additional residues of the sequence in the COOH-terminal direction) is as follows:*

Val	Gln	Leu	Ala	His	His	Phe	Ser	Glu	Ile	Glu	Ile	Thr	Leu	Ile
				5					10					15
Val	Phe	Gly	Val	Met	Ala	Gly	Val	Ile	Gly	Thr	Ile	Leu	Leu	Ile
				20					25					
Ser	Tyr	Gly	Ile	Arg	Arg	Leu	Ile	Lys	Lys					
				35↑					40					
				T										

In addition, all the chief lipids of the red-cell membrane are present in the chloroform-methanol extract of T(is), which quantitatively accounts for all of the lipid bound to the MN-glycoprotein [44].

---

*The amino acid sequence of the MN glycoprotein has recently been completed (M. Tomita and V. T. Marchesi, personal communication). One error appeared in the original sequence (residue 4, Pro → Ala). Several residues are still listed in the sequence as alternatives. The most likely in each case has been used in the sequence shown (at residue positions 6, 15, 16).

IV. TRANSVERSE LIPID-ASSOCIATING DOMAIN

A. Helicity of T(is) Peptide

Many earlier studies suggested that membrane proteins are highly helical [45-47]. In the MN-glycoprotein, the hydrophobic domain is the sole portion with a significant possibility of being alpha-helical. The NH_2-terminal domain, because of charge repulsion between sialic acid residues, and the C-terminal domain, because of the helix-breaking tendency of its prolines, are unlikely to have more than a trivial alpha-helical component.

Examination of the sequence of the 23 residue hydrophobic domain reveals that most of its residues are helix-inducing, according to the classification of Lewis and Scheraga [48]. In particular, there is a high content of leucine, suggested as the key residue involved in helix induction [49, 50], and an absence of proline.

A computer analysis by Robson and Pain [50] suggests that certain residues tend to promote helix formation in either an NH_2- or a COOH-terminal direction along the polypeptide chain from their location; glutamyl residues promote helix in a COOH-terminal direction and arginyl and lysyl residues in an NH_2-terminal direction. The nonpolar domain lies immediately COOH-terminal to two glutamyl residues (Residues 9 and 11) and NH_2-terminal to arginyl residues (Residues 35 and 36) and two lysyl residues (Residues 39 and 40). These same general conclusions hold also for the hydrophobic domain from the filamentous bacteriophage coat protein B [25, 26].

The NH_2-terminal tryptic peptide of MN-glycoprotein, $T(\alpha-1)$, is 34 residues long and contains 80% of the carbohydrate [40]. The COOH-terminal cyanogen bromide fragment C-2 of MN-glycoprotein forms a partial overlap with the hydrophobic domain [30]. The tryptic fragment T(is) contains the hydrophobic domain intact [39]. Circular dichroism (CD) spectra for the intact glycoprotein and the main carbohydrate-containing tryptic peptide, $T(\alpha-1)$, in aqueous solution, and the hydrophobic fragments T(is) and C-2 in trifluoroethanol (TFE), are shown in Figure 1. Percentage helix for the intact glycoprotein and $T(\alpha-1)$ in 0.1 M Tris-NaCl and the fragment C-2 and T(is) in TFE were determined by a three-component curve-fitting procedure described elsewhere [44]. These data indicate that the MN-glycoprotein, containing bound lipids in aqueous solution, has approximately 19% alpha-helix, and that the remaining is random structure [44, 51]. Recent CD data from another laboratory support this finding [52]. The hydrophobic domain of the MN-glycoprotein is composed of 23 amino acid residues, and is equal to 20% of the intact polypeptide chain. It is further evident that the hydrophobic domain represents 65% of the hydrophobic tryptic peptide T(is), 28% of the COOH-terminal cyanogen bromide fragment C-2, and none of the principal carbohydrate-containing tryptic peptide, the NH_2-terminal $T(\alpha-1)$. On the basis of curve fitting, the percentage of helix of each of the latter three peptides [84, 31, and 0, respectively] closely agrees with that portion of helix represented by the hydrophobic domain [44]. These data, together

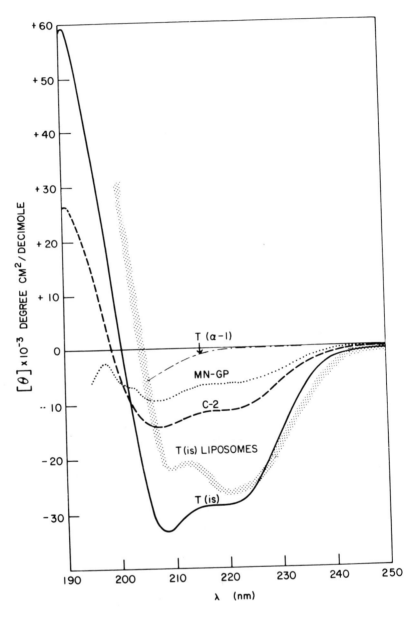

FIG. 1 Helicity of transverse lipid-associating domain from MN-glyco-protein. Circular dichroism spectra of T(α - 1) and MN-glycoprotein in 0.1μ Tris-NaCl, C-2 and T(is) in 2, 2, 2-trifluoroethanol and T(is) in egg lecithin liposomes.

with data published elsewhere concerning the relative helical stability of the hydrophobic domain [44, 51], suggest that this domain of the MN-glycoprotein is helical in the low dielectric environment of the membrane core, and composes the major helical portion of the glycoprotein. The 23-residue hydrophobic domain in the form of an alpha-helix would be 35Å long, which is the order of thickness, 33-40 Å [53], of the aqueous discontinuity of red-cell membranes.

The red-cell membrane appears to be composed of an asymmetric phospholipid bilayer [54, 55]. The inner half of the leaflet has a net negative charge on the basis of an asymmetric localization of phosphatidylserine to this half of the bilayer. A negative inner membrane surface would be complementary to the presence of 5 positively charged residues in a cluster at the presumably cytoplasmic end of the membrane-spanning 23-residue hydrophobic domain. By a similar agreement, the NH_2-terminal end of the hydrophobic domain contains two residues of glutamic acid, which could interact with the phosphatidylcholine residues, although the lipids of the outer surface presumably have a neutral net electrical charge. A probable function of these two collections of like-charged residues is to "lock" the MN-glycoprotein into the membrane. Alternatively, these domains may serve as recognition sites.

B. Linear Hydrophobic Sequences

If the hydrophobic domain of MN-glycoprotein is involved in protein-lipid interactions of the membrane, then its properties should in some manner be distinguishable from similar segments from non-membrane-associating protein. This hypothesis has been tested by computer analysis, described elsewhere [27]. The results of this study show that the 23-residue hydrophobic domain of MN-glycoprotein is distinguishable from virtually all hydrophobic domains of other proteins by its hydrophobicity relative to its length. The only other protein segments comparable to the hydrophobic domain of the MN-glycoprotein are the hydrophobic domains of the B coat protein of the filamentous bacteriophages (FV) discussed previously and the 15-residue polypeptide antibiotic gramicidin A.

C. Lipid Association of T(is) Peptide

1. Helicity

On the basis of the supposition that the membrane-associative properties of MN-glycoprotein reside in its 23-residue hydrophobic domain, and therefore, in the tryptic peptide T(is), studies were undertaken to examine the interaction of T(is) with hydrated phospholipid bilayers. The proposal that the hydrophobic domain is helical in situ is further supported by Figure 1, which shows that the T(is) polypeptide is approximately 75% alpha-helical

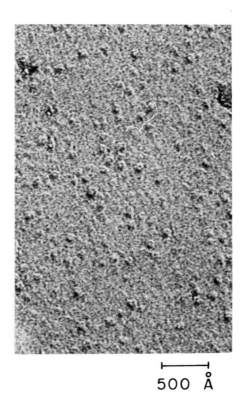

500 Å

FIG. 2 Self-association of transverse lipid-associating domain from
MN-glycoprotein. Freeze-fracture electron micrograph of T(is)-egg lecithin
complexes.

when associated with egg-lecithin liposomes [44, 56]. In addition, artificial
bilayers or black films can be formed from the T(is)-liposome complexes.
At a low ratio of T(is) to lecithin, the resistance of black films is decreased
significantly [57].

2. Freeze-Fracture Studies

    The nature of T(is)-egg lecithin complexes has been studied by freeze-
fracture electron microscopy [56]. Freeze-fracture of hydrated egg lecithin
multilamellar vesicles alone produces smooth fracture faces, representing
the hydrocarbon interior of the bilayer. The addition of T(is) to the liposomes
results in torus-shaped particles 80 Å in diameter (Fig. 2). It is assumed
that since these particles extend more than 15-20 Å above the surrounding
fracture face, they penetrate the bilayer completely.

The number of particles increases linearly with the addition of T(is); at a finite T(is) concentration, the curve extrapolates to zero particles [56]. This suggests a micelle-like phenomenon, in which at a critical concentration (the critical multimer concentration), T(is) prefers to associate with itself rather than with the surrounding phospholipids. From the slope of the curve, and from knowledge of the surface area occupied per phospholipid molecule (65 Å) in a bilayer, and an estimate of the surface area for each helical T(is) molecule, it is calculated that each particle represents a multimer composed of four or more T(is) molecules.

Below the critical concentration of T(is), monomers of the peptide can exist in the bilayer in two possible orientations, either forming an alpha-helix perpendicular to the hydrocarbon chains of the bilayer immediately below the polar head groups or forming an alpha-helix parallel to the hydro-carbon chains and spanning the aqueous discontinuity of the bilayer. As this critical concentration is exceeded, multimeric aggregation of T(is) occurs, producing intramembranous structures with defined toruslike shapes and a rotational symmetry 4-6. The size of these structures is independent of T(is) concentration. The topomolecular anatomy of the T(is) molecule is most compatible with the conclusion that the toruslike particles are formed of multimers of alpha-helical rods lying in parallel and spanning the aqueous discontinuity of the bilayer. A perpendicular orientation of the helix relative to the hydrocarbon chains in the middle of the bilayer is possible but is not compatible either with the torus shape or with the rotational symmetry of the multimers seen by freeze-fracture electron microscopy. Because these helixes therefore seem to transverse the bilayer in an orientation parallel to the hydrocarbon chains of the phospholipids, they are designated transverse lipid-associating domains. Evidence is presented in the following section that the plasma lipoproteins have helical lipid-associating regions with an orientation opposite that proposed for transverse domains, that is, perpendicular to the fatty acyl chains of the phospholipid structures.

V. PROTEINS OF THE PLASMA LIPOPROTEIN

The plasma lipoproteins are macromolecular associations of lipid with protein that are in essence "soluble" in aqueous media such as blood plasma and extracellular fluid. Plasma lipoproteins serve both as substrates for enzymes involved in lipid metabolism and as vehicles for the transport of lipid. For a recent review of the structure and function of the plasma lipo-proteins, the reader is referred to Morrisett et al. [3]. The human blood plasma lipoproteins have been classified into four main groups, as follows: chylomicrons, lipoproteins of very low density (VLDL), low-density lipo-proteins (LDL), and high-density lipoproteins (HDL). The composition of these classes has been summarized elsewhere [58]. The protein components (apoproteins) of the plasma lipoproteins can be freed of their lipid by extrac-tion in organic solvents. The apoproteins have been separated by a variety of techniques, usually in urea or sodium decyl sulfate [59, 60]. The amino acid sequences for four of the apolipoproteins of the human plasma lipoproteins are known [61-65]. Two of these apolipoproteins (apoC-I and apoC-III) are predominantly found in VLDL but also are present in HDL, and two (apoA-I and apoA-II) are found in HDL. The availability of these amino acid sequences is important because the information for the lipid-binding properties of these proteins is encoded within their sequences. However, in contrast to integral membrane proteins, that is, the erythrocyte MN-glycoprotein, the plasma apoproteins have no long hydrophobic sequences.

VI. SURFACE LIPID-ASSOCIATING DOMAIN

A. Amphipathic Helixes

One clue to the mechanism of lipid association in the plasma lipoproteins is the finding that lipid-free apoproteins when recombined with phospholipid undergo a change in protein conformation, as measured by circular dichroism, that corresponds to an increase in alpha-helical structure. Consideration of this fact led us recently to propose a specific topomolecular model to explain the interaction of apoproteins from VLDL and HDL with the lipid of their respective blood plasma lipoprotein particles [66]. The model predicts that specific phospholipid-associating sites along the polypeptide chain of the apoproteins are alpha-helical. Furthermore, there is a specific surface topographical distribution of the polar and nonpolar residues of the chain. It is proposed that these helixes, on the basis of their topography, are complementary for the surface of hydrated phospholipid aggregates. Each helix is divided into polar and nonpolar faces in an amphipathic manner, as illustrated in Figure 3A. Further, there is a specific distribution of charged residues along the polar face. The negatively charged residues invariably occur in a narrow longitudinal strip down the center of the polar face and the positively charged residues occur along the interfacial edge between the polar and nonpolar faces. Of particular interest in this distribution is the occurrence of topographically close complementary ion pairs (four in the example shown in Fig. 3A). Eighteen regions with this topographical feature occur in the amino acid sequences of the four apoproteins whose sequences are known. These predicted helical lipid-associating domains are consistent with the total helicity and location of known lipid-binding sites for each apolipoprotein [67].

Surface distribution of charged residues relative to the nonpolar face (Fig. 3B, upper and middle) is exactly complementary to the molecular topography of phospholipid molecules such as phosphatidylcholine and phosphatidylethanolamine. It is proposed that these complementary amphipathic helical regions associate with hydrated phospholipid aggregates by half-burying themselves at the interface between the hydrocarbon chains and the polar head groups of the phospholipid aggregates. The lower part of Figure 3B

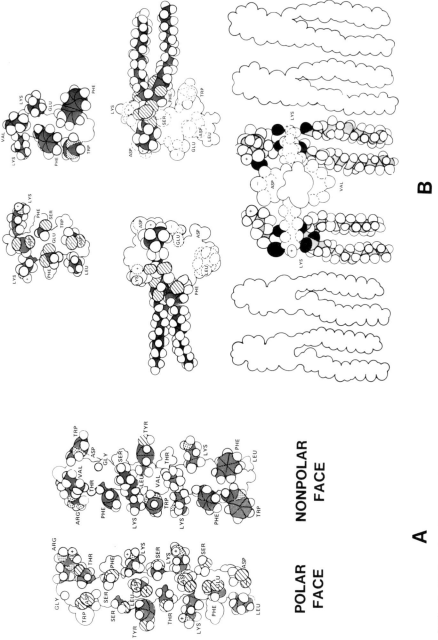

FIG. 3 Molecular topography of surface lipid-associating domain from Apo LP-CIII. A. Residues 40-67 built as an alpha helix with CPK-space filling molecular model. B. Residues 56-67 (upper), showing complementarity to phosphatidylcholine (middle) and in association with phosphatidylcholine water-hydrocarbon interface (lower).

shows the amphipathic helix viewed down its length from the NH_2-terminal end. In this model, the helix lies perpendicular to the water-hydrocarbon surface of the fatty acyl chains of phospholipid structures, and for this reason, the lipid-binding regions within the plasma lipoproteins VLDL and HDL are designated surface lipid-associating domains.

B. Computer Analyses of Occurrence and Properties

Partly because of the description by Perutz et al. [68] of helical regions within globular proteins that have nonpolar faces (representing edges buried within the protein interior), it was of interest to determine the frequency of occurrence of amino acid sequences in all classes of proteins that fitted the criteria of amphipathic helixes as described. On the basis of a plane of symmetry defined by the negatively charged residues at the center of the polar face, a computer program was constructed to select amino acid sequences that fitted the desired criteria. With this program, a datum tape containing known protein sequences was searched [69]. A minimal residue length of 11 was set and the limits of each acceptable segment were determined by the occurrence of residues at forbidden positions along the sequence relative to the plane of symmetry presented by an amphipathic helical structure. Sixty-five amino acid sequences containing at least two ion pairs were found that fitted the criteria for amphipathic helixes. Those with three or more ion pairs are shown in Table 1. While many presumably non-lipid-binding proteins do contain regions of sequence that fit these criteria, 35% of the 65 regions are in lipid-binding proteins. This is in spite of the fact that these proteins represent less than 2% of sequenced homologous protein classes. This means that known lipid-binding proteins are enriched in hypothetical amphipathic helixes by a factor of approximately 20 over the remaining, and presumably non-lipid-binding, proteins.

If the general features of the amphipathic lipid-associating model are correct, a switch in the position of the positive and negative residues would seemingly be unfavorable, since this would put them adjacent to like charges in the phospholipid structure. This assumption has been supported by the following computer studies. When the position of the charged residues in the computer search program were switched (so that positive residues lay centrally in the polar faces), numerous sequences capable of forming reversibly polarized amphipathic helixes were found in a wide variety of proteins. The reversed "helixes" were different from the complementary "helixes" in two ways [69].

1. The reversed "helixes" contained considerably fewer topographically close ion pairs, their distribution fitting a random distribution, whereas the original complementary amphipathic helixes were considerably enriched over random in three and especially four ion-pair-containing helixes (Table 2).

2. By a hydrophobicity scale originally designed for studying the hydrophobic domain of the MN-glycoprotein [27] (Trp, +6.5; Phe, +5.0; Ile, +5.0;

TABLE 1

Computer Selected Amphipathic Sequences

Ion pairs	Protein	Hydrophobicity index of nonpolar face	Residue length	Residue position
4	Enterotoxin B (S. aureus)	5.0	15	71–85
	Apo LP–CIII (Human)	4.6	28	40–67
	Myoglobin (Human)	4.6	15	38–52
	Apo LP–AI (Human)	4.2	26	8–33
	Apo LP–CI (Human)	4.2	21	33–53
	Amyloid A (Human)	3.5	26	1–26
	Serum albumin (Human)	3.4	20	4–23
3	Actin (Rabbit)	4.8	11	206–216
	Apo LP–AII (Human)	4.7	21	10–30
	Lactalbumin (Bovine)	4.6	12	6–17
	Enterotoxin B (S. aureus)	4.4	15	217–232
	Trypsin inhibitor (Soybean)	4.4	15	106–120
	Apo LP–CI (Human)	3.8	12	18–29
	Alcohol dehydrogenase E (Horse)	3.6	14	222–235
	Keratin, low–sulfur fraction (Sheep)	3.6	14	64–77
	Lactoglobulin (Bovine)	3.5	14	130–143
	Apo LP–AI (Human)	3.1	14	131–144
	Growth hormone (Bovine)	3.1	15	99–114
	Amyloid A (Human)	1.7	22	53–74

TABLE 2

Occurrence of Multiple Ion Pairs in Amphipathic Sequences

No. of ion pairs	Number of amphipathic sequences		Number of reversely polarized sequences	
	Actual	Random*	Actual	Random*
≥ 1	649	...	581	...
2	124	92	77	83
3	13	8	5	8
4	7	0	0	0

*Calculated from the probability of occurrence of a second set of ion pairs within a given sequence length (one chance in seven), calculated in turn from the percentage occurrence of each of the charged residues [76]. Since the occurrence of each ion pair requires an additional 5 residues in the sequence, the final probability distribution depends on the occurrence of longer sequences and therefore is progressively truncated as one goes beyond 2 ion pairs.

Tyr, +4.5; Leu, +3.5; Val, +3.0; Met, +2.5; Pro, +1.5; Ala, +1.0; His, +1.0; Thr, +0.5; Gly, 0; Cys, 0; Ser, -0.5; Gln, -1.0; Asn, -1.5), the reversed sequences have nonpolar faces with significantly lower mean hydrophobicity indexes per residue (HI) on average (HI = 2.5) than the amphipathic sequences have (HI = 3.0).

The most remarkable aspect of these data is that the seven sequences that contain four ion pairs (Table 1) have extraordinarily hydrophobic nonpolar faces (mean HI = 4.2). This value is higher than the HI's of the membrane-associating hydrophobic domains of the MN-glycoprotein and the two filamentous bacteriophage coat proteins from ZJ-2 and FD, with HI's of 2.62, 2.86, and 2.91, respectively [27]. Five of the seven sequences, including amyloid A (see below), are from proteins known to bind lipids. The results are not quite so clear-cut for those eleven sequences containing three ion pairs (Table 1) although they have significantly hydrophobic nonpolar faces (HI = 3.8), and several are from known lipid-binding proteins.

On the other hand, one might postulate that to replace the specifically placed charged residues in the complementary amphipathic helix with polar residues such as serine and threonine also would be less favorable for association with phospholipid structures due to the low degree of hydration of hydroxyl groups compared with charged groups. Again, this assumption has been supported by computer studies. The search program was modified so that the polar residues on the polar face had a random distribution. Again, the average hydrophobicity of the nonpolar faces of the potential helixes located by the program was significantly decreased by this modification over the hydrophobicity of the original complementary amphipathic helixes [69].

C. Amyloid A

With a list of amino acid sequences that meet the criteria of complementary amphipathic helixes and gathered from all classes of proteins available, one test of the amphipathic model would be to select a protein containing a potential lipid-binding sequence (a protein not known to be a lipid binder) and show convincingly that the protein is, in fact, a lipid-binding protein.

One such protein is amyloid A (Table 1), a pathologically occurring protein isolated from tissue deposits in human patients with secondary amyloidosis of unknown origin and function [70]. This protein contains two regions (with 4 and 3 ion pairs) of amino acid sequence that fit the criteria of amphipathic helixes. When amyloid A provided by Dr. George Glenner of the NIH was tested, it fulfilled three criteria for lipid binding [71]. These are (1) a phosphatidylcholine vesicle-amyloid complex can be isolated by ultracentrifugation between d 1.063-1.210 g/ml; (2) there is a marked increase (by a factor of approximately 4) in alpha-helicity as measured by circular dichroism with the addition of phosphatidylcholine vesicles to amyloid A; (3) when amyloid A is added to sonicated phosphatidylcholine vesicles, stacked discs are formed, and can be seen by negative-stain electron microscopy.

VII. THERMODYNAMIC IMPLICATIONS

An informal comparison of the thermodynamic properties of the transverse-versus-surface lipid-associating domains (LAD) should be useful to understanding the binding mechanisms involved. The transverse LAD is insoluble in water but soluble in the hydrocarbon interior of the hydrated phospholipid bilayer. This suggests that there is a large increase in negative free energy as the transverse LAD goes from water to a hydrated phospholipid bilayer. This does not occur spontaneously, however, but requires the expenditure of energy; that is, the bilayer structure must be disrupted by solubilization of phospholipid in ethanol [56]. These observations are summarized in Figure 4. The high-energy barrier from water to phospholipid bilayer

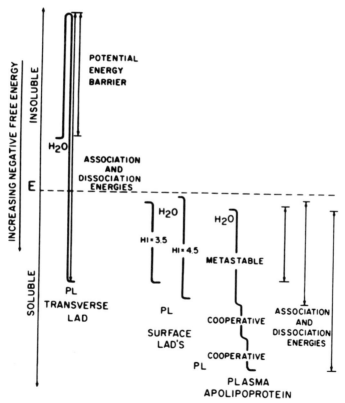

FIG. 4 Thermodynamics of movement of transverse and surface lipid-associating domains from water to phospholipid. Informal energy diagram of transverse and surface lipid-associating domains and intact plasma apolipoprotein.

solubility represents the energy required to force the highly charged ends of the transverse LAD, represented by the tryptic peptide T(is), through the low dielectric interior of the bilayer membrane. This is a highly unfavorable situation and accounts for the height of the barrier. The configuration of this energy curve is such that the transverse LAD once present within a hydrated bilayer is quite stable and requires the disruption of the structure of the bilayer for its removal, for example with detergents or organic solvents.

On the other hand, the surface LAD is partially soluble in water. Because of the removal of the hydrophobic residues of the nonpolar face of the surface LAD from aqueous solution and into the interfacial hydrocarbon region of a hydrated bilayer, there is an increase in negative free energy in associating the surface LAD with the bilayer. This association occurs spontaneously, suggesting there is little or no potential-energy barrier in going from aqueous to hydrated bilayer solubility. This means that the surface LAD, in general, should be removable from a hydrated bilayer to water without disrupting the

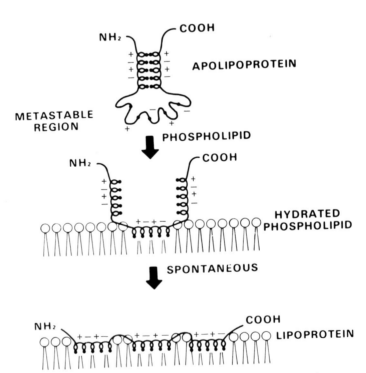

FIG. 5 Model for association of intact plasma apolipoprotein with the polar-nonpolar interface of phospholipid.

structure of the bilayer. It seems likely that the surface LAD would tend to be reversible in its association with phospholipids. It seems quite clear that hydrophobicity of the nonpolar face would be directly related to the tightness of lipid association. These observations are summarized in Figure 4, and in Figure 5 have been combined into a model for the mechanism of lipid association of surface LAD-containing proteins such as the plasma lipoproteins. At least one potential surface LAD in each delipidated apolipoprotein is assumed to exist in a nonhelical metastable (partially soluble) conformation (a hydrophobic patch on the protein surface) until exposure to phospholipid. On exposure to phospholipid, this metastable region seeks its lowest free energy by forming a surface LAD at the water interface with hydrated phospholipid vesicles. Other surface lipid-associating domains (already of helical conformation), whose nonpolar faces have been sequestered from water by interacting with one another, are now free to interact with the hydrated phospholipid. This model is consistent with the observation that tryptophan residues exposed to solvent in delipidated apo-CI are buried in a nonpolar environment when the apolipoprotein is recombined with phospholipid [72].

VIII. IMPLICATIONS FOR MEMBRANE STRUCTURE

A. Transverse Domain

The evidence presented here suggests that in vitro and possibly in vivo [56] the hydrophobic domain of the MN-glycoprotein forms oligomeric helical structures (80 Å in diameter) that transverse the aqueous discontinuity of hydrated phospholipid bilayers with the helixes parallel to the hydrocarbon chains of the phospholipid molecules. Constructing a space-filling molecular model from the known amino acid sequence in the vicinity of the hydrophobic domain of MN-glycoprotein provides some insight into possible mechanisms involved in the intrabilayer self-association of helical segments of the tryptic peptide T(is). The surface topography of this model (Fig. 6) is remarkable in that the helix is divided into two faces. One face contains bulky hydrophobic residues. The opposite face contains, in its central portion, a collection of neutral nonbulky residues, primarily glycyls and alanyls but also one hydroxy amino acid residue. This bisection of the surface topography of the hydrophobic domain from the MN-glycoprotein and the surface LAD's from the plasma lipoproteins suggest that these may be extreme examples of a general design for lipid-associating domains of lipoproteins.

A space-filling molecular model constructed as an alpha helix from the known amino acid sequence of the hydrophobic domain of the B coat protein from the filamentous bacteriophage ZJ-2 [25, 26] provides support from such a general model. As shown in Figure 6, this hydrophobic domain is also roughly divided into two faces, one having bulky hydrophobic residues (A) and the opposite face having a central neutral groove, composed primarily of glycyls, that runs the length of the face (B). This is compatible with the

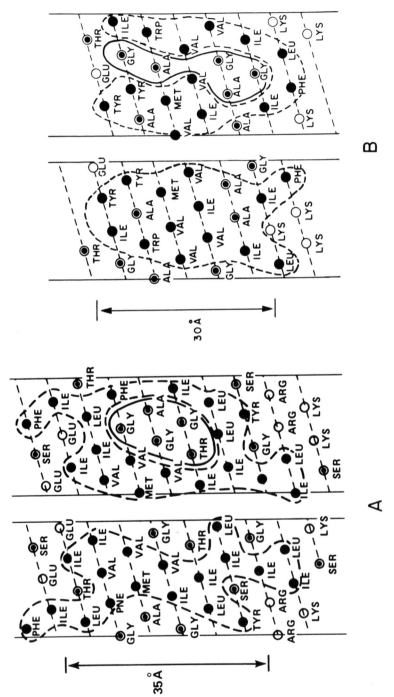

FIG. 6 Alpha-helical net of transverse lipid-associating domains of (A) MN-glycoprotein and (B) B coat protein from filamentous bacteriophages ZJ-2. ●, Hydrophobic, ⊙, neutral and 0, charged amino acid residues.

observation that the coat protein forms dimers when associated with deter-gents [73, 74]. There is no experimental evidence that the hydrophobic domain of the B coat protein is alpha-helical, although, as will be discussed later, the region almost certainly must be either alpha-helical or beta-helical within a bilayer.

If one calculates HI's for the neutral and hydrophobic halves of the MN-glycoprotein and ZJ-2 LAD's (1.2, 4.3 and 1.3, 4.5 respectively), one finds that although their overall hydrophobicities are less than the mean of nonpolar faces of the amphipathic helixes with four ion pairs (HI = 4.2), the HI's of the hydrophobic faces of the three are comparable.

B. Surface Domain

We propose the following general model for lipid-associating domains of lipoproteins. The transverse and surface LAD's are similar in that both are alpha-helical and involve collections of extremely hydrophobic amino acid residues with an HI of approximately 4.0. They differ in that the surface LAD contains one face that not only is less hydrophobic than the opposite face but has charged amino acid residues distributed in a complementary arrangement relative to the charged head groups of phospholipid molecules. Transverse LAD's can be classified into two distinct types. One is that in which the alpha helix is featurelessly hydrophobic, for example, gramicidin A (total HI = 3.6) [27]. In this case, there would be no tendency for adjacent transverse LAD's within bilayers to associate with one another as oligomers. The second type of transverse LAD contains two distinct faces, one that is extremely hydrophobic and another that is essentially neutral but may con-tain hydroxy amino acids (and possibly charged amino acids). Protein-protein association to form intramembraneous structures occurs between the neutral edges (association edges) of these self-associating transverse LAD's.

C. Mechanism for Self-Association of Transverse Domains

Interactions between lipid-solubilized helical polypeptide chains along neutral edges can be rationalized as follows. Spontaneous transient electric fields arise at every point in a molecular structure due to the transitory fluctu-ations of electric charge. Interactions of these transient electric fields pro-duce the Van der Waals force. Since the electron fluctuation is proportional to the absorption of light by the particular molecular structure [75], hydro-carbons that have a low light dispersion (that is, are colorless and trans-parent) would be expected to be relatively poor producers of Van der Waals interactions. It therefore follows that the hydrophobic faces of the transverse LAD's would have little tendency to interact in the low dielectric environment of the membrane core, but the neutral faces, with higher electron mobility, would have quite significant Van der Waals interactions. Further, because of electron fluctuation synchrony, like structures associate best, that is, neutral faces with neutral faces and hydrophobic faces with the multitude of hydrocarbon chains of the bilayer. Once a transmembrane oligomeric structure is assembled, then a second, more powerful force might come into play, the formation of a water bridge in the midportion of the structure.

IX. SUMMARY

We propose that the following general principles apply to a wide variety of membrane or plasma lipoproteins. Lipid-associating domains of lipoproteins will consist of relatively short polypeptide segments. One likely reason for restriction in length of these domains would be the instability of very long domains during biosynthesis of the lipoproteins. These lipid-associating domains, if they are longer than a few residues, will be invariably alpha-helical or helical in the sense that a beta-pleated sheet is a helix with a twofold rotational symmetry. The tremendous increase in negative free energy achieved by formation of intramolecular or intermolecular hydrogen bonds produces the helical structures. Otherwise, polypeptide chains longer than a few residues with free-backbone polar amino and carbonyl groups would be insoluble within the low dielectric environment of the membrane. These lipid-associating domains will interact with lipid primarily through hydrophobic interactions although electrostatic interactions will occur at the water-lipid interface in a topographically distinct fashion, depending on whether the domain is transverse or surface-oriented. Complex intramembranous structures can be built up from interactions between short polypeptide domains of the transverse variety. These interactions may be intermolecular associations of numerous monomers or intramolecular associations within a single protein. In general, this interaction will be between associating edges composed of neutral and hydroxy amino acid residues. On the other hand, there will be no tendency for protein-protein interactions of surface-oriented lipid-associating domains per se. Protein-protein interactions between plasma apolipoproteins in situ, for example, must involve regions of the protein that are topographically distinct from the lipid-associating domains.

ACKNOWLEDGMENTS

We acknowledge contributions by D. G. Dearborn, R. J. Feldmann, T. Gulik-Krzywicki, L. D. Kohn, and C. Sardet to portions of this work, and wish to thank A. M. Gotto for helpful criticisms. R. L. J. is an established investigator of the American Heart Association. This work was partially supported by HEW grants DE-02670, HL-14194, HL-03435/34, and HL-16512/01.

REFERENCES

1. L. Sachs, M. Inbar, and M. Shinitzky, in Control of Proliferation in Animal Cells, ed. B. Clarkson and R. Beserga. New York: Cold Spring Harbor Laboratory, 1974, p. 283.
2. G. L. Nicolson , in Control of Proliferation in Animal Cells, ed. B. Clarkson and R. Beserga. New York: Cold Spring Harbor Laboratory, 1974, p. 251.
3. J. D. Morrisett, R. L. Jackson, and A. M. Gotto, Ann. Rev. Biochem., 44, 183 (1975).
4. H. Davson and J. F. Danielli, in The Permeability of Natural Membranes, 2nd ed., London: Cambridge University Press, 1952.
5. D. A. Haydon, in Permeability and Function of Biological Membranes, ed. L. Bolis, A. Katchalsky, R. D. Keynes, W. R. Loewenstein, and B. A. Pethica. Amsterdam: North Holland Publishing Co., 1970, p. 185.
6. V. Luzzati, T. Gulik-Krzywicki, A. Tardieu, and F. Reiss-Husson, in The Molecular Basis of Membrane Function, ed. D. C. Tosteson. Englewood Cliffs, N. J.: Prentice-Hall, 1969, p. 79.
7. Y. K. Levine, A. I. Bailey, and M. H. F. Wilkins, Nature, 220, 577, (1968).
8. D. M. Engelman, J. Mol. Biol., 58, 153 (1971).
9. L. Spatz and P. Strittmatter, Proc. Nat. Acad. Sci. U.S., 68, 1042 (1971).
10. F. S. Mathews, F. S., M. Levine, P. Argos, Nature New Biol., 233, 15 (1971).
11. N. C. Robinson and C. Tanford, Biochemistry, 14, 369 (1975).
12. R. A. Cone, Nature New Biol., 236, 39 (1972).
13. M. Chabre, A. Cavaggioni, H. B. Osborne, T. Gulik-Krzywicki, and J. Olive, FEBS Letters, 26, 197 (1972).
14. K. Hong and W. L. Hubbell, Biochemistry, 12, 4517 (1973).
15. J. K. Blasie, personal communication.
16. M. S. Bretscher, J. Mol. Biol., 59, 351 (1971).
17. G. Fairbanks, T. L. Steck, and D. F. H. Wallach, Biochemistry, 10, 2606 (1971).
18. J. A. Kant and T. L. Steck, Nature New Biol., 240, 26 (1972).
19. I. Yu and T. L. Steck, Fed. Proc., 33, Abs. 1740 (1974).
20. K. Wang and F. M. Richards, Fed. Proc., 33, Abs. 424 (1974).
21. Z. I. Cabantchik and A. Rothstein, J. Membrane Biol., 10, 331 (1972).
22. M. K. Ho and G. Guidotti, J. Biol. Chem., 250, 675 (1975).
23. P. Pinto da Silva and G. L. Nicolson, Biochem. Biophys. Acta, 363, 31 (1974).
24. H. Garoff and K. Simons, Proc. Nat. Acad. Sci. U.S., 71, 3988 (1974).
25. D. T. Snell and R. E. Offord, Biochem. J., 127, 167 (1972).
26. F. Asbeck, K. Beyrenther, H. Kohler, G. Wettstein, and G. Braunitzer, Hoppe-Seyler's Z. Physiol. Chem., 350, 1047 (1969).

27. J. P. Segrest and R. J. Feldmann, J. Mol. Biol., 87, 853 (1974).
28. D. A. Marvin and B. Hohn, Bacteriol. Rev., 33, 1972 (1969).
29. R. E. Webster and J. S. Cashman, Virology, 55, 20 (1973).
30. J. P. Segrest, I. Kahane, R. L. Jackson, and V. T. Marchesi, Arch.
     Biochem. Biophys., 155, 167 (1973).
31. M. S. Bretscher, Nature New Biol., 231, 229 (1971).
32. R. Sarges and B. Witkop, J. Amer. Chem. Soc., 86, 1862 (1964).
33. D. W. Urry, M. C. Goodall, J. D. Glickson, and D. F. Mayers, Proc.
     Nat. Acad. Sci. U.S., 68, 1907 (1971).
34. W. R. Veatch, E. T. Fossel, and E. R. Blout, Biochemistry, 13, 5249
     (1974).
35. M. Ohnishi and G. D. Urry, Science, 168, 1091 (1970).
36. A. I. McMullen, D. I. Marlborough, and P. M. Bayley, FEBS Letters,
     16, 278 (1971).
37. R. J. Winzler, in Red Cell Membranes: Structure and Function, ed.
     G. A. Jamieson and T. J. Greenwalt. Philadelphia: J. P. Lippincott,
     1969, p. 157.
38. A. Morawiecki, Biochim. Biophys. Acta, 83, 339 (1964).
39. J. P. Segrest, R. L. Jackson, V. T. Marchesi, R. B. Guyer, and
     W. Terry, Biochim. Biophys. Res. Commun., 49, 961 (1972).
40. R. L. Jackson, J. P. Segrest, I. Kahane, and V. T. Marchesi, Bio-
     chemistry, 12, 3131 (1973).
41. S. Grefrath and J. A. Reynolds, Fed. Proc., 33, Abs. 1738 (1974).
42. H. Furthmayr, M. Tomita, and V. T. Marchesi, Fed. Proc., 34,
     Abs. 1879 (1975).
43. T. W. Tillack, R. E. Scott, and V. T. Marchesi, J. Exper. Med.,
     135, 1209 (1972).
44. J. P. Segrest, in Mammalian Cell Membranes, ed. G. A. Jamieson
     and A. M. Robinson. London: Butterworths, 1977.
45. J. Lenard and S. J. Singer, Proc. Nat. Acad. Sci. U.S., 56, 1828
     (1966).
46. A. S. Schneider, M. T. Schneider, and K. Rosenheck, Proc. Nat.
     Acad. Sci. U.S., 66, 793 (1970).
47. D. W. Urry, L. Masotti, and J. R. Krivacic, Biochim. Biophys. Acta,
     241, 600 (1971).
48. P. N. Lewis and H. A. Scheraga, Arch. Biochem. Biophys., 144, 576
     (1971).
49. P. Y. Chou, M. Wells, and D. W. Fasman, Biochemistry, 11, 3029
     (1972).
50. G. Robson and R. H. Pain, Nature New Biol., 238, 107 (1972).
51. J. P. Segrest and L. D. Kohn, Proceedings of the 21st Colloquium,
     Brugge, Belgium, Protides of the Biological Fluids, ed. H. Peeters.
     Oxford: Pergamon Press, 1973, p. 183.
52. R. V. Decker and K. L. Carraway, Biochim. Biophys. Acta, 386, 52
     (1975).

53. J. B. Stamatoff, S. Krimm, and N. R. Harvie, Proc. Nat. Acad. Sci. U.S., 72, 531 (1975).
54. M. S. Bretscher, Nature New Biol., 236, 11 (1972).
55. M. S. Bretscher, J. Mol. Biol., 71, 523 (1972).
56. J. P. Segrest, T. Gulik-Krzywicki, and C. Sardet, Proc. Nat. Acad. Sci. U.S., 71, 3294 (1974).
57. E. J. A. Lea, G. J. Rich, and J. P. Segrest, Biochim. Biophys. Acta, 382, 41 (1975).
58. R. I. Levy, D. W. Bilheimer, and S. Eisenberg, in Plasma Lipoproteins, ed. R. M. S. Smellie. London and New York: Academic Press, 1971, p. 3.
59. W. V. Brown, R. I. Levy, and D. S. Fredrickson, J. Biol. Chem., 245, 6588 (1970).
60. A. Scanu, J. Toth, C. Adelstero, S. Koga, and E. Stiller, Biochemistry, 8, 3309 (1969).
61. H. B. Brewer, S. E. Lux, R. Ronan, and K. M. John, Proc. Nat. Acad. Sci. U.S., 69, 1304 (1972).
62. H. B. Brewer, R. Shulman, P. Herbert, R. Ronan, and K. Wehrly, Advan. Exptl. Biol. and Med., 26, 280 (1972).
63. R. Shulman, P. Herbert, K. Wehrly, B. Chesebro, R. I. Levy, and D. S. Fredrickson, Circulation, 45, II-246 (1972).
64. R. L. Jackson, J. T. Sparrow, H. N. Baker, J. D. Morrisett, O. D. Taunton, and A. M. Gotto, J. Biol. Chem., 249, 5308 (1974).
65. H. N. Baker, T. Delahunty, A. M. Gotto, and R. L. Jackson, Proc. Nat. Acad. Sci. U.S., 71, 3631 (1974).
66. J. P. Segrest, R. L. Jackson, J. D. Morrisett, and A. M. Gotto, FEBS Letters, 38, 247 (1974).
67. R. L. Jackson, J. D. Morrisett, A. M. Gotto, and J. P. Segrest, Mol. Cell. Biochem., 6, 43 (1975).
68. M. F. Perutz, J. C. Kendrew, and H. C. Watson, J. Mol. Biol., 13, 669 (1965).
69. J. P. Segrest and R. J. Feldmann, Biopolymers, in press.
70. G. G. Glenner, W. D. Terry, and C. Isersky, Seminars in Hematology, 10, 65 (1973).
71. J. D. Morrisett, J. S. K. David, H. J. Pownall, and A. M. Gotto, Biochemistry, 12, 1290 (1973).
72. R. L. Jackson, J. D. Morrisett, J. T. Sparrow, J. P. Segrest, H. J. Pownall, L. C. Smith, H. F. Hoff, and A. M. Gotto, J. Biol. Chem., 249, 5314 (1974).
73. S. Makino, J. L. Woolford, C. Tanford, and R. E. Webster, J. Biol. Chem., 250, 4327 (1975).
74. J. L. Woolford and R. E. Webster, J. Biol. Chem., 250, 4333 (1975).
75. V. A. Parsegian, in Annual Review of Biophysics and Bioengineering, Vol. 2, ed. L. J. Mullins, W. A. Hagins, and L. Stryer. Palo Alto: Annual Reviews, 1973, p. 3
76. C. R. Reeck and L. Fisher, Int. J. Peptide Protein Res., 5, 109 (1973).

Chapter 3

LIPID PROPERTIES AND LIPID-PROTEIN INTERACTIONS

Giorgio Lenaz

Istituto di Biochimica
Facoltà di Medicina e Chirurgia
University of Ancona
Italy

ABBREVIATIONS

ANS, 1-anilinonaphthalene-8-sulfonate; AS, 12(9-anthroyl) stearic acid; CD, circular dichroism; CMR, ^{13}C magnetic resonance; CoQ, coenzyme Q; DANS-Cl, 1-dimethylaminonaphthalene-5-sulfonyl chloride; DCCD, dicyclohexyl carbodiimide; DMR, deuterium magnetic resonance; DSC, differential scanning calorimetry; DTA, differential thermal analysis; DTT, dithiothreitol; EFA, essential fatty acids; ESR, electron spin resonance; F_1, "factor 1" of oxidative phosphorylation: the oligomycin-insensitive ATPase; IR, infrared;

MW, molecular weight; NEM, N-ethyl maleimide; NMR, nuclear magnetic resonance; NPN, N-phenyl naphthylamine; NS, doxylstearic acid; ORD, optical rotatory dispersion; OSCP, oligomycin-sensitivity-conferring protein; PA, phosphatidic acid; PC, phosphatidyl choline; PE, phosphatidyl ethanolamine; PG, phosphatidyl glycerol; PI, phosphatidyl inositol; PMR, proton magnetic resonance; PS, phosphatidyl serine; PTS, phosphoenol pyruvate glucose phosphotransferase; SDS, sodium dodecyl sulfate; SR, sarcoplasmic reticulum; TEMPO, 2,2,6,6-tetramethylpiperidine-1-oxyl; T_f, temperature of onset of phase separation (separating fluid from mixed phase); T_s, temperature of completion of phase separation (separating solid from mixed phase); 9-VA, 9-vinyl anthracene.

I. INTRODUCTION

Protein-lipid interactions play a key role in the structural and functional properties of membranes. These interactions can be classified as two types. There are specific interactions between proteins and lipids that affect the structural and functional properties of both components. At the same time the lipid as a bulk phase is important in orienting proteins to the compartments separated by any membrane.

As introduction to the many results now available on protein-lipid interactions, it is important to define what we mean by a membrane protein and also to review briefly the properties of lipids in a bilayer, and as they exist in membranes, for these properties can and do modulate the properties of the proteins in contact with lipid.

As described in the first chapter, it is now conventional to separate membrane proteins into two classes [1, 2]. Intrinsic, or integral, membrane proteins are those proteins that penetrate the lipid bilayer partially and even completely and have primarily hydrophobic interactions with lipids. Extrinsic membrane proteins are loosely associated with the surface of the membrane by predominantly hydrophilic or electrostatic interactions. As I shall discuss, both types of protein affect lipids and are affected by association with them.

II. SYSTEMS USED TO STUDY THE PROPERTIES OF LIPIDS AND THEIR INTERACTIONS WITH PROTEINS

The properties of lipids and their interaction with proteins have been studied in native membranes and in a variety of model systems among which only lamellar structures (i.e., bilayers) should be rigorously included. The studies with lipid monolayers, however, have contributed to such an extent to knowledge of membrane structure and in particular of lipid-protein interactions that they are here considered as half-membranes maintaining the molecular relations found in bilayer membranes. As for bilayer systems, many technical approaches are available, including single bilayers separating

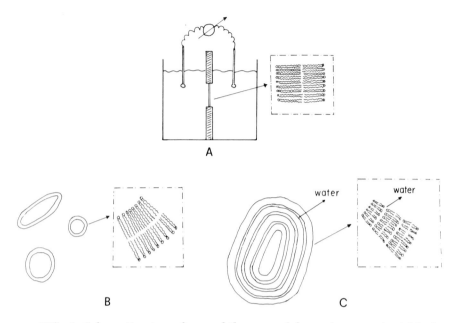

A

B   C

FIG. 1 Schematic view of some bilayer model membranes. A. A black
lipid membrane. B. Single bilayer vesicles. C. A multibilayer liposome.
Arrows point to magnified details of the bilayer systems.

two aqueous phases ("black" lipid membranes), lamellar multibilayers such
as the liposome systems (or "banghosomes"), and lamellar single-bilayer
vesicles (Fig. 1).

A. Lipid Monolayers

Theoretical principles and experimental techniques on monolayers have been
given by Cadenhead [3], Kézdy [4], and Papahadjopoulos [5], among others.
Phospholipids can be spread at an air-water interface to form an insoluble
monolayer in which the molecules are oriented perpendicular to the plane of
the surface, with the polar groups facing the water phase and the hydrocarbon
chains directed into the air phase. The classical technique for making monolayers involves spreading the phospholipids in a trough with a moving barrier
for sweeping the surface and compressing the film. Amphipathic molecules
will form monomolecular films that can be compressed to different extents
when the surface area is changed by simply moving the barrier. The property
most usually measured experimentally is the surface pressure π, defined as
the difference between surface tension of pure water γ_0 and the surface tension
of the monolayer-covered surface γ:

$$\pi = \gamma_0 - \gamma$$

Since phospholipids and other surfactants lower the surface tension of water, π has a positive value measured in dynes/cm. The magnitude of π varies with the surface concentration of the surfactant molecules and depends on temperature and nature of the molecules and in general on all factors affecting their cohesion. It is possible either to measure surface pressure under different conditions or to make force-area curves, that is, to subject the monolayer to different compressions and to measure the area per molecule of the monolayer. Different physical states have been described (from gas to solid until the collapse of the monolayer). Different phospholipids show different force-area curves; at a given temperature, saturated and long-chain phospholipids are more condensed than unsaturated and short-chain phospholipids, which occupy a larger area (Å/molecule). Also the polar head will influence the packing of the monolayer.

Other conditions that can be studied are surface potential (arising from the permanent dipoles or charges of the monolayer surface), surface viscosity, and also surface activity.

Proteins or other molecules can be added to the subphase, and changes in the above-mentioned physical properties can be measured so that interpretations at the molecular level can be obtained [6, 7], such as ionic interactions or penetration. Manipulations on the surface (use of proteolytic or lipolytic enzymes) can also be used to allow molecular interpretations.

B. Black Lipid Membranes

When an amphipath above the transition temperature is smeared across a small hole joining two aqueous compartments, a bimolecular film that separates the two compartments is formed. Formation of the film can be followed visually by appearance of a black spot, which in a variable time extends to the whole film. These "black" lipid membranes are widely used as model membranes [5, 8-10]. The only prerequisite for a membrane-forming solution is that an amphipathic compound (e.g., phospholipid) and a neutral hydrocarbon solvent (e.g. n-decane) be present. Thickness measurements show that black membranes approach the theoretical thickness of a bimolecular layer. The hydrocarbon solvent complicates the bilayer picture and makes these membranes unphysiological at least in this respect.

The best-studied properties of a black membrane are its electrical characteristics: electrical capacitance (averaging 0.38 μF/cm^2) and electrical resistance. The electrical resistance for bilayers ranges from 10^6 to 10^9 $\Omega \cdot$cm^2 [11], in contrast with the lower resistance in biological membranes (10^2 to $10^5 \Omega \cdot$cm^2). The large resistance of pure lipid bilayers is compatible with their very low permeability to cations. The most likely origin of this barrier is the large energy required to bring ions from the aqueous phase into the low-dielectric-constant membrane interior formed by the nonpolar fatty acyl chains. Indeed, the magnitude of observed bilayer conductances is consistent with values calculated for a 50-Å-thin membrane having the properties of a bulk hydrocarbon phase [12].

Other measurements on bilayers include optical reflectance and direct electron microscopy.

Adding to one compartment compounds such as peptides, proteins, and drugs may modify the electrical properties of bilayers, and this has been the most widely used method of dealing with protein-lipid interactions in black lipid films. Large increases in conductance are generally interpreted as involving penetration of the film by the peptide molecules, with formation of channels across the membrane between the two aqueous phases. Stepwise discrete conductance increases provide evidence for the view that proteins induce polar channels across lipid bilayers.

Bilayers having different compositions on the two sides have been obtained by causing two lipid monolayers with different composition to interact [13]. Such bilayers are ideal for studying the molecular asymmetry of biological membranes, since proteins can be included in one or the other of the two interfacing monolayers separately.

C. Oriented Lipid Multibilayers

Successive layers of lipids can be deposited on glass plates by repeated dipping into monomolecular films at an air-water interface [14]. Different techniques are now available to form oriented multibilayers [15]. Films are formed either by filling the flat area of quartz ESR cells with the lipid solution and drying the solvent; or by drying liposomes on a microscope cover glass, after which the films are hydrated with a known percentage of water. Alternatively, dried lipids and water are mixed together and placed between glass plates; motion of one plate imparts a shearing force and orients the lipids into multibilayers parallel to the glass plates [16].

Multibilayers are suited for X-ray diffraction [17, 18] and particularly for ESR spin labeling, in which measurement can be made as a function of the angle between the magnetic field and the plane of the multibilayers [19-21]; analysis of a large number of spectra taken at different angles gives a much higher probability that the model for spin-probe behavior is unambiguous.

D. Bilayer Vesicles and Liposomes

When amphipathic lipids are allowed to swell in water above the transition temperature, they form closed onionlike lamellar structures (myelin figures or liposomes) [22-24] that consist of stacked lamellae of phospholipids in bilayer configuration, with water filling the spaces between the lamellae. Each lamella is formed of a continuous permeability barrier [25], and the efflux rates of incorporated isotopic tracers can be determined by dialysis or passage through a gel filtration column, or by using ion-specific electrodes. Liposomes have advantages over black lipid membranes, since they are better defined chemically (no decane or other solvent present) and present in higher quantity; but electrical properties cannot be measured.

Ultrasonic irradiation of liposomes breaks up the coarse particles into small vesicles, eventually to a homogeneous population of small single-bilayer vesicles of 200–500-Å diameter [26, 27]. The particle weight of the vesicles is 1.5×10^6 to 2.1×10^6, corresponding to 1.9×10^3 to 2.7×10^3 molecules per vesicle. Electron spin resonance studies with spin labels (see later) have shown that 65% of the phospholipid molecules are present in the external monolayer of the small vesicles with their very high curvature [28].

Phospholipid vesicles are osmotically sensitive to salts and small molecules. They swell in hypotonic solutions and shrink in hypertonic solutions. Optical methods can be applied in studying the osmotic behavior and water permeability in multilayered liposomes. Diffusion rates for ions through phospholipid vesicles have been studied, and the effects of lipid composition and additions to the medium on these rates have been investigated [5]. Specific examples of protein-liposome interaction and physical studies on liposomes and reconstituted membranes will be developed in the further sections of this chapter.

III. LIPID PROPERTIES AND TECHNIQUES USED IN THEIR STUDY

The most characteristic property of amphipathic lipids is that they undergo a thermotropic phase transition at well-defined temperatures. Since lipid fluidity is considered one of the main aspects of membrane structure and is largely affected by proteins, it seems pertinent to consider here an up-to-date outlook of lipid fluidity, of the methods used to assess fluidity, and how fluidity is affected by endogenous and exogenous factors. A detailed review on perturbation of membrane fluidity has been published elsewhere [29]. In this section we shall also consider specific aspects of the mobility of membrane components (diffusion, rotation, and the like).

A. Lipid Fluidity and Phase Separations

Raising the temperature of a pure crystalline lipid induces an endothermic transition at a specific temperature, where the hydrocarbon chains of the component fatty acids "melt" and become liquidlike in mobility, while the polar moieties are still in a rigid, quasi-crystalline structure [30-33].

At constant pressure, the free-energy change is zero and the entropy increase (disorder) of melting is accomplished at the expense of an enthalpy change. The transition can be detected by a wide range of techniques that "probe" the thermodynamic, geometric, and kinetic changes of the fatty acid components at the transition. A serious ambiguity in studies of membrane fluidity is that different probes do not necessarily detect the same types of physical changes. As discussed elsewhere [29], the terms mobility, fluidity, disorder, and so forth are not given the same meaning by investigators using the different techniques. For this reason, it is appropriate to review briefly the common methods for studying lipid fluidity in bilayers and membranes.

1. Differential Scanning Calorimetry

Calorimetric techniques are best suited for studying the "melting" phenomena [34, 35]. In differential thermal analysis (DTA), the sample and a reference material are heated at the same rate. The difference in temperature remains zero or constant until a phase change occurs in the sample, at which time the differential temperature increases, with emergence of a peak; the direction of this peak indicates whether the reaction is exothermic or endothermic. A better method for quantitative analysis is differential scanning calorimetry (DSC), in which the temperatures of sample and reference material are kept equal, and what is measured is the differential power needed for maintaining a sample temperature equal to the reference temperature; this power is directly related to the heat absorbed during an endothermic transition (Fig. 2).

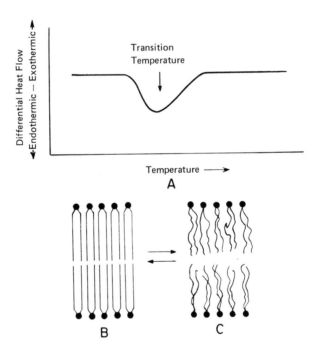

FIG. 2 Thermotropic transition of amphipathic lipids. The diagram (A) shows an idealized calorimetric scan of amphipathic lipids, indicating the endothermic transition from the crystalline to the liquid-crystalline phase. The lower scheme shows the state of the lipids at temperatures (B) lower and (C) higher than the transition temperature.

The endothermic transitions are sharp for homogeneous lipids (same class and same fatty acid content). The transition temperature is decreased by hydration of the lipids [31] until a constant value is reached at 40% water content. The bound water within these limits does not show a phase change and is presumed to be "iceberg" water.

The transition temperature depends on both the polar and the apolar phospholipid moieties. The effect of fatty acid composition on the transition temperature is obvious, considering the importance of Van der Waals attractions among the fatty acid chains. The more unsaturated the lipid, the lower the transition temperature, since cis double bonds decrease chain cohesion. On the other hand, increasing chain length will enhance the interaction energy among chains and the transition will occur at a higher temperature [35]. It is less directly obvious why different lipid classes, even those having the same fatty acid composition (e.g. dipalmitoyl PC and dipalmitoyl PE), have different transition temperatures; in this case the nature and interactions involving the polar head must affect the hydrocarbon chains to different extents. In general, PE has a higher transition temperature compared with its PC analog, due to the bulky properties of the choline headgroup, which decrease cohesion of the hydrocarbon chains: for example, dimyristoyl PE melts at 45 °C, whereas dimyristoyl PC melts at 25 °C [36].

The phase behavior of phospholipids may be modified by exogenous and endogenous agents. (I shall report in detail the effects of proteins and cholesterol on the transitions in a later section.) However, it has been shown also that changes in the ionic environment of a bilayer may significantly affect the transitions. The cation Ca^{2+} and other cations increase significantly the transition temperature of anionic phospholipids; UO_2^{2+} also affects zwitterionic lecithin [37]. An increase in the temperature of transition is also induced by lowering the pH of the medium, an indication that protonation of anionic groups in phospholipids induces a better packing of the fatty chains [38, 39]. It is not within the scope of this review to report the alterations of lipid phase transitions induced by pharmacologically active compounds [cf. 40].

For binary mixtures of synthetic phospholipids, different situations may occur [35, 37]. For lipids having similar fatty acid composition, only one transition is observed, which is intermediate between the transitions of the pure components. For lipids with differing fatty acid content, however, when the chain length difference is above four methylene groups, two transitions become apparent. Even when the fatty acid composition is the same, two transitions may also occur with lipids belonging to different classes. Sometimes mixing of this kind results into broad endotherms.

In the temperature region between the two endothermic peaks, or within the broad single peak, solid and liquid phases coexist in the same bilayer, the solid phase containing an excess of the component having the higher transition temperature [41]. Phase separation is now recognized in most lipid mixtures, although other methods besides DSC are available to detect this phenomenon. Phase diagrams may be built from the calorimetric scans, as well as from the behavior of spin labels (see later).

Natural lipid mixtures (usually containing several lipid classes and a wide variety of fatty acid species within the same class) show, as it may be expected, a very wide endothermic peak, which is centered near 0 °C in the case of liver mitochondrial phospholipids [42]. Such a large range of melting temperatures must result from the combined thermotropic behavior of the different component lipids. It is reasonable for phase separation to occur and for solid and fluid patches to coexist in the same bilayer (or membrane). For lipid mixtures (e.g. zwitterionic plus anionic lipids), exogenous agents (Ca^{2+}, pH) may induce phase separation. This effect has been proved also by other methods and will be discussed later.

Differential scanning calorimetry also gives information on the quantitative aspects of the thermal transitions. The area under the calorimetric peak will be proportional to the enthalpy of transition. Calculating the thermodynamic limits in thermotropic transitions is important in defining the effects of such agents as cholesterol, peptides, and drugs.

For a first-order transition at constant pressure, the free-energy change is zero and the latent heat equals the enthalpy change ΔH, and $\Delta H = T \Delta S$. The heat absorbed (positive ΔH) is used to increase the disorder of the hydrocarbon chain (positive ΔS). Quantitative values of the heat involved in the melting processes have been given by Phillips et al. [43]. Also, Chapman [35] should be consulted for thermodynamic and theoretical geometric aspects of the transitions.

2. X-Ray Diffraction

Phase transitions are also detectable by X-ray diffraction [44, 45]. As Cain et al. [45] have pointed out, X-ray diffraction alone cannot distinguish between the ensemble average of a frozen statistically disordered structure and a dynamic structure whose time average is identical to the ensemble average of the frozen structure. Luzzati and his coworkers [32, 46-49] have shown that several mesomorphic phases, which are not liquid-crystalline, are characterized by various extents of long-range and short-range disorder and are not comparable with a true crystalline state. To gain information about molecular motion in a structure, correlations may be attempted between X-ray diffraction and other techniques. Nevertheless, studies of pure phospholipid bilayers below and above the transition temperature have revealed two well-defined patterns: crystalline packing is characterized by a sharp Bragg reflection at 4.15 Å, while at 4.5 Å a broad maximum with considerable spreading occurs above the transition. Moreover, above the transition, the hydrocarbon core of the bilayer thins dramatically. In heterogeneous lipids the transition between the two states is gradual, and reflects phase separation. The breadth of the transitions will depend on the partition coefficient of the mixed lipids between the ordered and disordered domains [44].

3. Electron Microscopy

Like X-ray crystallography, electron microscopy detects the geometry of lipids on the two sides of a transition. Freeze–fracture (and freeze-etching) electron microscopy is the only microscopic technique that gives meaningful details on the chemical architecture of a membrane [50, 51]. Freeze–fracture electron microscopy is clearly able to distinguish lipids in the liquid–crystalline state from lipids in crystalline arrangement. Electron micrographs show wide bands with a spacing of 192 Å when the sample is

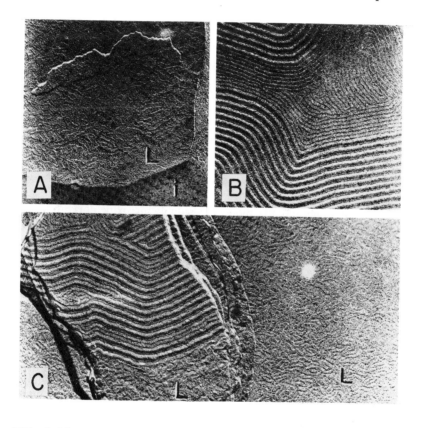

FIG. 3 Platinum–carbon replicas of liposome fracture for 50/50 mole percentage mixtures of dielaidoyl and dipalmitoyl PC quenched from various temperatures. Magnification ×81,000. A. Liposome quenched from 36 °C (fluid). B. Liposome quenched from 10°–11 °C (gel). C. Liposome quenched from 30 °C, showing appreciable areas of gel phase in equilibrium with fluid lipid. i, ice; L, lipid. Reproduced from Grant et al. [53], with kind permission of Elsevier Publishing Company.

quenched (rapidly frozen) from a temperature below the phase transition, whereas smooth indistinct areas are present when the sample is quenched from above the transition [52, 53]. In the regions corresponding to phase separation, clear patches of rigid lipids and of fluid domains exist within the same microscopic field, giving a visual indication of the phase separation phenomenon [53, 54] (Fig. 3).

4. Spin-Labeling

The use of electron spin resonance (ESR) of paramagnetic probes (spin labels) is one of the most important spectroscopic techniques in the study of biomembranes. All spin labels are nitroxide derivatives in which the $N \rightarrow O$ group contains an unpaired electron that renders the molecule paramagnetic. The spin label introduced into interesting sites of membranes or membrane components absorbs electromagnetic radiation in the presence of an external magnetic field, and the interaction of the unpaired electron with nuclear spin produces a <u>hyperfine splitting</u> of the absorption spectrum with three lines at increasing magnetic field. The shape of the spectrum reflects the orientation and motion of the spin label and the polarity of its environment [55–57].

Spin labels are nowadays very popular as probes of lipid mobility in bilayers and membranes. Different categories of spin labels have been used for this purpose (Table 1).

One type of spin label is the water-soluble nitroxide derivatives such as TEMPO (2,2,6,6-tetramethylpiperidine-1-oxyl) and related compounds [58]. TEMPO has a higher partition coefficient for fluid than for rigid lipids and has been used as a sensitive probe for <u>phase separation</u> in lipid mixtures. The upper field line of the ESR spectrum has a different position in polar and nonpolar environments and a splitting is evident when the label is present in both environments in the same sample. By plotting the ratio of the two peak heights against temperature (or the reciprocal of temperature in an Arrhenius plot), two discontinuities are observed in binary mixtures such as those described for DSC studies, which have been associated with the onset (T_f) and the completion (T_s) of phase separation. The temperature region between the two "breaks" corresponds to the temperature range within which solid and fluid regions coexist. Phase diagrams of T_f and T_s against the ratio of the two components define three regions: the <u>solidus</u> region (S phase), the <u>fluidus</u> region (F phase), and in between, a region of heterogeneous state separated from the other regions by lines joining the experimentally determined T_f and T_s (Fig. 4).

Another important aspect related to phase separation has been revealed by TEMPO. Even for a pure lipid like dioleyl lecithin [59], the partition of TEMPO has shown the formation of quasi-crystalline clusters at 30 °C, well above the phase transition (-22 °C). This phenomenon is common for many liquids. Only at high temperatures do the molecules exist in the true

TABLE I

Selected Examples of Spin Labels Used in Membrane Structure Studies

1 — Partition Labels

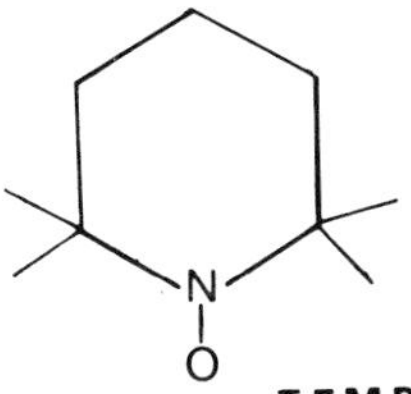

2 — Fatty Acid Labels

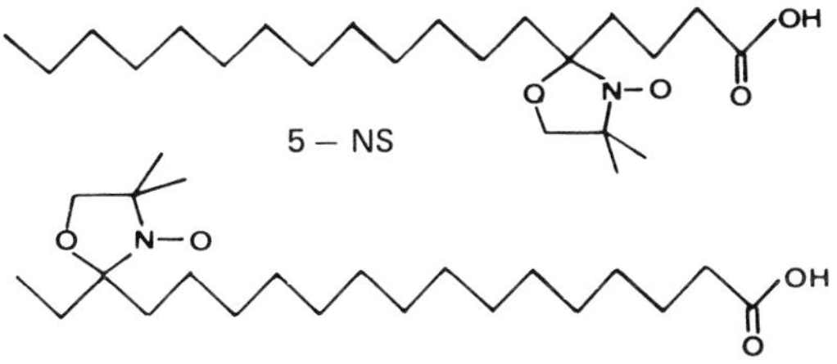

5 — NS

16 — NS

TEMPO

3 — Phospholipids Labels

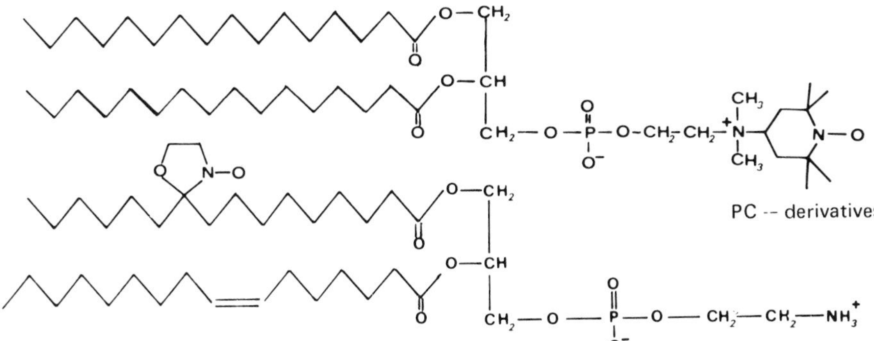

PC -- derivatives

PE — derivatives

4 — Steroid Labels

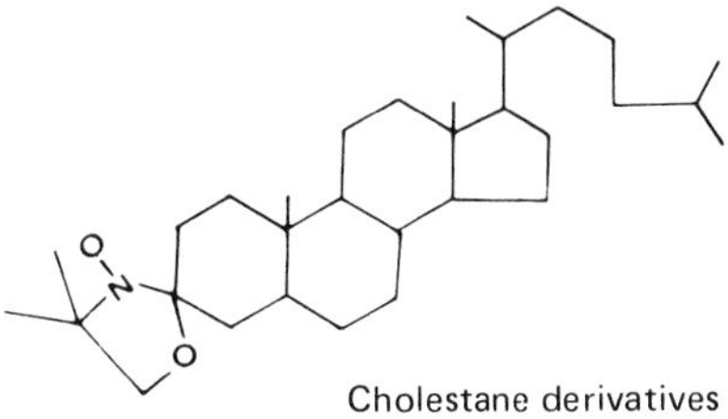

Cholestane derivatives

5 — Protein Labels

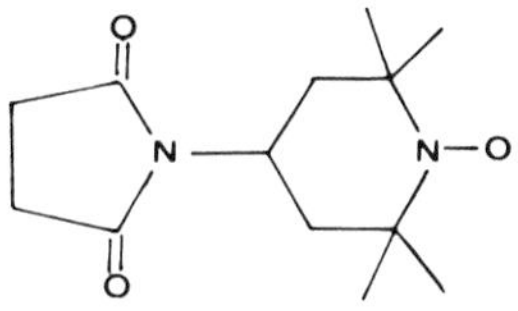

Maleimide derivatives

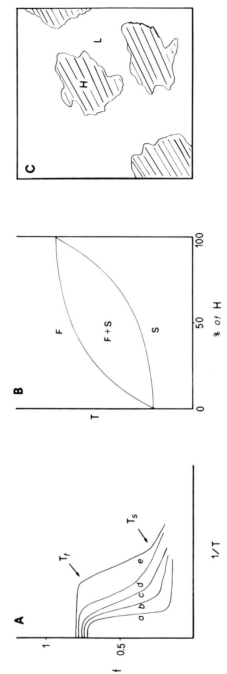
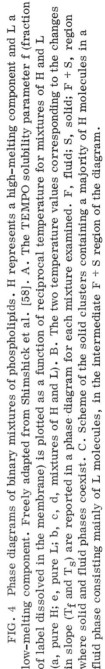

FIG. 4 Phase diagrams of binary mixtures of phospholipids. H represents a high-melting component and L a low-melting component. Freely adapted from Shimshick et al. [58]. A. The TEMPO solubility parameter f (fraction of label dissolved in the membrane) is plotted as a function of reciprocal temperature for mixtures of H and L (a, pure H; e, pure L; b, c, d, mixtures of H and L). B. The two temperature values corresponding to the changes in slope (T_f and T_s) are reported in a phase diagram for each mixture examined. F, fluid; S, solid; F + S, region where solid and fluid phases coexist. C. Scheme of the solid clusters containing a majority of H molecules in a fluid phase consisting mainly of L molecules, in the intermediate F + S region of the diagram.

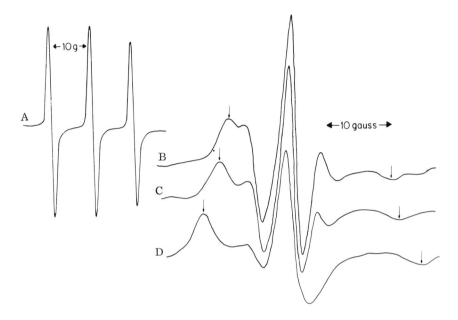

FIG. 5 ESR spectra of 5-doxylstearic acid in different systems, showing different extents of immobilization. A. In water. B. In phospholipid vesicles. C. In mitochondrial membranes. D. In lipid-depleted mitochondria. Arrows point to the hyperfine splitting extrema.

monomeric state. If the lifetime of the clusters is long enough, they behave as whole particles and are detected as separate phases.

A second class of spin labels includes fatty acid derivatives such as those of stearic acid, which have a nitroxide at different position in the hydrocarbon chain (5, 12, 16 being the most used). The shape of the paramagnetic spectrum is very sensitive to probe rotational mobility, described by the rotational correlation time τ_c:

$$\tau_c = 6.5 \times 10^{-10} \, W_0 \left(\sqrt{\frac{h_0}{h_{-1}}} - 1 \right)$$

where W_0 is the width of the medium-field line, and h_0, h_{-1} refer to the heights of the medium and upper-field lines. Practically, τ_c is valid for times lower than 10^{-9} sec [60], but indications of bilayer fluidity are often given by empirical conditions such as the h_0/h_{-1} ratio, or the distance in gauss between the hyperfine splitting extremes $(2T_\parallel)$ (Fig. 5).

The order parameter S accurately describes the state of the lipid chains:

$$S = \frac{T_{\parallel} - T_{\perp}}{T_{zz} - 0.5(T_{xx} + T_{yy})} \cdot \frac{a}{a'}$$

where T_{zz}, T_{xx}, and T_{yy} are the intrinsic (rigid lattice) hyperfine principal values, $T_{\parallel}$ and $T_{\perp}$ are the values observed when the nitroxide is located in the experimental system, and a and a' are the isotropic parts of the hyperfine interaction in the rigid and fluid matrix respectively. The values $T_{\parallel}$ and $T_{\perp}$ are often easily calculated from the ESR spectra. The previous equation can be recalculated as

$$S_n = 0.568 \frac{T_{\parallel} - T_{\perp}}{a'}$$

where $a' = (1/3)(T_{\parallel} + 2T_{\perp})$.

Computer simulation of the motion of the lipid hydrophobic chains has been attempted to obtain quantitative data of bilayer viscosity from strongly immobilized nitroxides [10, 61, 62].

The lipid mobility decreases with decreasing temperatures, and discontinuities are found in the Arrhenius plots of the correlation times or other motion conditions [63]; the breaks appear related to T_f and T_s of phase separation. Raison and McMurchie [64] have found two breaks for the motion of spin-labeled fatty acids in mitochondrial membranes, one in the upper and the second in the lower range of the calorimetric transition. It appears, therefore, that these labels also detect phase separation. The reason why fatty acid spin labels and TEMPO give similar information may be in their preferential affinity for fluid areas in bilayers when fluid and solid areas are present at the same time [65]. Such preferential distribution, however, results in extrusion of the labels from solid into fluid bilayer areas, limiting the information furnished by these labels to the mobility of components in fluid areas only.

Sterol spin labels, like the N-oxyl-4',4'-dimethyloxazolidine derivative of cholestane-3-one, appear suited for investigating absolute average fluidities of a bilayer, since they do not appear to be segregated into fluid areas. Butler et al. [66] have obtained experimental and theoretical spectra for the cholestane probe in lipid mixtures having different proportions of saturated and unsaturated acids; they found good agreement, in contrast with the large deviations from theory, in the case of fatty acid labels when fluid and solid areas coexist.

Spin labels have revealed a very important aspect of fluidity in bilayers. A fluidity gradient has been found with increased mobility from the polar headgroups towards the terminal methyl groups, by using stearic acid labels that have the nitroxide at varying distances from the carboxyl groups and

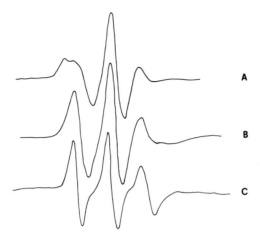

FIG. 6   The fluidity gradient observed with stearic acid spin labels in phospholipid vesicles. A. 5-Doxylstearic acid. B. 12-Doxylstearic acid. C. 16-Doxylstearic acid.

hence at varying depths in the bilayer [55, 67-70] (Fig. 6). There is an immobilizing effect of the polar headgroups on the nearest methylene groups. However, the fluidity gradient detected by spin labels has not been fully confirmed by other methods such as deuterium magnetic resonance (see later). It appears that spin labels behave as impurities, since the bulky nitroxide induces perturbation in the surrounding regions, as detected by monolayer studies [71]. Moreover, the exact location of a fatty acid label is not known with certainty and may depend on the ionization state of the headgroup [7]. This particular drawback can be circumvented by using spin-labeled phospholipids, synthesized in vivo by supplementing spin-labeled fatty acids to fatty-acid-requiring microorganisms [73, 74].

   Spin labels have been used extensively to examine the effects of endogenous or exogenous perturbing agents. The effect of Ca^{2+} on phase separation in mixed bilayers of PS and PC has been studied [75] by taking advantage of the line broadening due to the spin-spin interactions that occur when the spin labels are brought together by two-dimensional phase separation. Ca^{2+} chelation segregates solid PS aggregates from a fluid phase consisting of PC alone. Similar clustering is observed in PA-PC bilayers, but not for other mixtures [76].

   Using spin labels to detect such phenomena as lateral and transverse mobility of lipids will be discussed later. The effect of proteins and cholesterol on spin-label motion will also be described later.

   A vast literature is accumulating on the effects that drugs (especially narcotics and anesthetics) exert on lipid mobility, but a full review is beyond the scope of this chapter. The reader may find pertinent literature in other reviews [29, 77].

5. Fluorescent Probes

When a light-excited electron returns to the ground state from the lowest excited state, light is emitted, a phenomenon called fluorescence. The quantum yield (the fraction of quanta emitted) depends on the nature of the lowest excited state, and also on the nature of environmental molecules or groups that cause collisional quenching of fluorescence. Polarization of fluorescence is also a function of the nature (viscosity) of the solvent that affects the freedom of rotation of the fluorescent molecule. For reviews cf. Refs. 78 and 79.

Only recently, however, have fluorescent molecules found wide applications as probes of fluidity (as well as polarity) in bilayers and membranes. It is convenient to discuss briefly the spectral properties of a classic probe such as ANS (1-anilinonaphthalene, 8-sulfonate). This substance is strongly fluorescent in hydrophobic media, with a maximum near 475 nm, but its fluorescence is quenched in water with a shift of emission maximum to about 520 nm. ANS is located in the polar region of the lipid bilayer [80] and thus probes the glycerol region. It is therefore used as a surface probe [81]. Being an amphipathic molecule, however, ANS is stabilized hydrophobically, and its interaction with a bilayer is best described as a partition phenomenon from water to a more hydrophobic medium. The pattern of a double reciprocal plot of fluorescence against membrane concentration strongly suggests a partition phenomenon according to the following equation:

$$\frac{1}{F} = \frac{W_W}{PF^0W_P} + \frac{1}{F^0}$$

where F = fluorescence, W_W = weight of the water phase, W_P = weight of the membrane phase, P = partition coefficient (expressed as the ratio of probe concentration per unit weight of membrane phase and water phase), and F^0 = fluorescence corresponding to the total amount of probe present, that is, maximal fluorescence at infinite membrane concentration. The plot of $1/F$ vs $1/W_P$ is linear in the hypothesis of a partition phenomenon and the intercept at the ordinate gives the value of $1/F^0$, which is a function of the quantum yield of the ANS "bound" to the membrane when all ANS added is "bound" (Fig. 7). From the slope of the plot it is possible to calculate the partition coefficient of ANS between membrane and water [82]. In this respect, the effect of salts is highly suggestive. Salts increase the partition of ANS into octanol. The extent of this effect depends on the nature of the salt, and chaotropic anions like SCN^- [83] have the lowest effect. Since chaotropic agents decrease the polarity of water, the partition of ANS in octanol must be a function of the difference in hydrophobicity between the two phases. Interestingly, the same linear dependence holds for the "binding" of ANS to

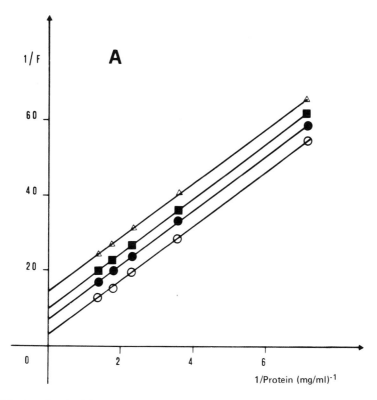

FIG. 7 The double reciprocal plot of ANS fluorescence vs membrane concentration. The abscissa is the reciprocal of protein concentration in mito-chondrial membranes. The four straight lines indicate four experimental conditions leading to decreased F^0 (n-butanol addition) while the partition coefficient (from the slope) is unchanged (unpublished studies).

a membrane, and analogous differences exist among the effects of different salts [82, 84]. Membrane binding of ANS must therefore be a function of the difference in hydrophobicity between water and membrane, and the effect of salts in enhancing ANS binding is not to be considered merely a charge effect.

ANS has mainly been used as a polarity probe, but its quantum yield is sensitive to the viscosity of its microenvironment [85] and it has been used to detect phase changes in membranes [81] and in general, membrane fluidity. The quantum yield of ANS fluorescence increases with decreasing temperature and therefore with lipid mobility in a fluid membrane. At the transition, however, a large decrease of fluorescence ensues, owing to poor partitioning into solid lipid phases [35]. This large change is useful for defining phase transition temperatures of membranes.

TABLE II

Structure of Some Fluorescent Probes

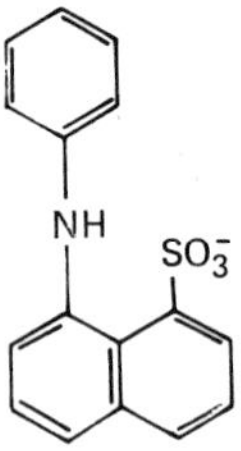

ANS

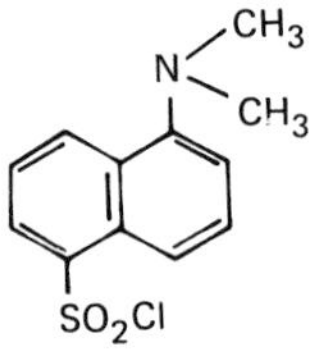

Dans-Cl

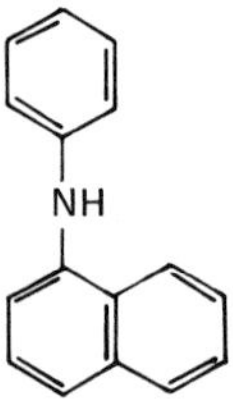

NPN

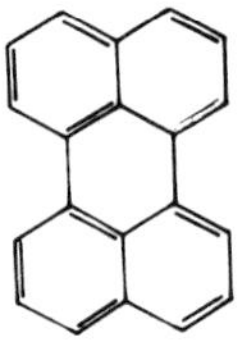

Perylene

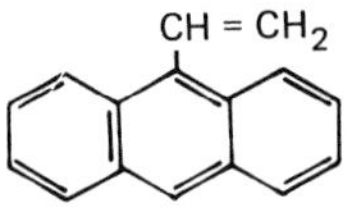

9-VA

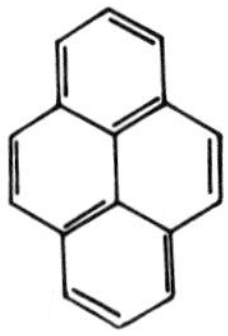

Pyrene

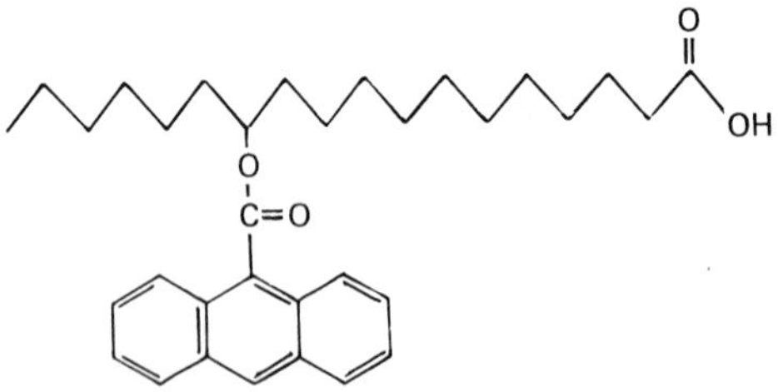

AS

Other fluorescent probes, including the amphipathic 12-(9-anthroyl)-stearate (AS), contain a fluorophore that buries deeply into the bilayer, and is therefore a probe of membrane core mobility [79, 86].

Other kinds of fluorescent probes are hydrophobic molecules located in nonpolar regions of bilayers [87], and provided that their spectral properties are sensitive to the microviscosity of their environment, they can be used as fluidity probes. The polarization of the fluorescence of perylene or anthracene derivatives is directly proportional to the viscosity of the bilayer core [88-90] and slope discontinuities in temperature dependence have been used to probe phase transitions.

Träuble and Eibl [91] found that phase transitions detected with the fluorescent probe N-phenyl-naphthylamine (NPN) are induced at constant temperature by changing the ionic environment of bilayers. A decrease of pH and Ca^{2+} addition both increase the transition temperature, while monovalent cations lower the transition temperature. Phase separation at constant temperature induced by slight changes of the ionic environment may have important implications in such functional phenomena as nerve transmission.

The formation of pyrene-excited dimers (excimers) has also been used to study lipid viscosity [87, 92, 93]. Table 2 gives the structures of some of the widely used fluorescent probes.

A criticism that can be advanced against fluorescent probes is that they (as spin labels) are foreign molecules that may perturb the bilayer.

Intrinsic fluorescence of protein chromophores (tyrosine, tryptophan) may be used in the case of natural and artificial membranes containing proteins [78]. The fluorescence of tyrosine, in contrast to tryptophan, is relatively insensitive to the polarity of solvent.

6. Nuclear Magnetic Resonance

Nuclear magnetic resonance (NMR) has been used extensively to probe the physical state of lipids in bilayers and membranes [35, 78, 94, 95]. Any nucleus with a nonzero magnetic moment will interact with electromagnetic radiation in the presence of an external magnetic field and absorb energy. It is possible to study selected nuclei independent of others (e.g. ^1H, ^2H, ^{13}C, ^{15}N, ^{31}P), and NMR will theoretically give information about the environment and molecular freedom of most of the atoms present in the structure of a membrane. So far, proton magnetic resonance (PMR) has been the most widely used.

A variety of methods are available for NMR studies. The most common method for obtaining NMR spectra is to use a spectrometer operating at fixed frequency (e.g. 60, 100, 220 MHz) while the external magnetic field is changed. Different nuclei at a given frequency will absorb at different values of magnetic field intensity. In addition, the local magnetic field for a given nucleus is modified by local molecular shielding effects leading to chemical shifts. The sensitivity increases with external field strength.

Various pulse techniques are available that can measure relaxation properties of the nuclei following a pulse of external radiation. The lifetime of the spin states is described by the spin-lattice relaxation time T_1, which is the time necessary for the populations of the two spin states to come to a new equilibrium in a pulse experiment. The time T_1 is one of the main factors contributing to linewidth of an NMR absorption. The value T_1 increases with temperature and is inversely proportional to the rotational correlation time τ_c, since nuclei in a molecule relax more efficiently by decreasing their tumbling rate; τ_c is directly related to viscosity of the medium.

The second important determinant of the linewidth is low-frequency dipole interactions between neighboring nuclei; the effect of molecular motion is to time-average the angular dependence of the low-frequency dipole interactions and then to narrow the linewidths.

It is clear then that in a phospholipid or membrane system, increase in chain motion will produce a narrowing of the linewidth with a considerable fall at the transition temperature, where molecular motion almost averages to zero the magnetic dipole-dipole interactions.

A complication of NMR is the dependence of resolution of the spectra of phospholipids on sonication. When a phospholipid-water system is examined by PMR, a broad spectrum is obtained, with the exception of the $N^+(CH_3)_3$ group protons of choline in lecithin. Sonication gives rise to high-resolution spectra with clear $(CH_2)_2$ signals from the fatty acid chains [96]. It is not yet fully resolved whether sonication affects the bilayer structure with modifications of molecular motion, or only breaks the system into small particles that have higher tumbling rates as a whole and reorient to average out dipolar interactions [97, 98]. It is clear from the geometry of the small vesicles that differences in packing may cause greater mobility in the bilayer of sonicated vesicles [99]. Recently, Lichtenberg et al. [100], using vesicles of different sizes, have presented evidence for the view that sonication disrupts the molecular packing of the chains.

Carbon-13 NMR is becoming of wider interest, because of certain advantages over PMR (e.g. less dipolar broadening); CMR studies have confirmed the indications given by PMR [35].

Deuterium magnetic resonance using phospholipids with deuterated fatty acid derivatives is able to probe the environment of the fatty chains without causing the same perturbation of environment that spin labels do. Seelig and coworkers [101-105] have confirmed by DMR that a fluidity gradient exists from the surface to the core of the bilayer, but it is not so evident and gradual as ESR indicated (Fig. 8). The difference has been ascribed to the perturbing effect of the nitroxides.

7. Infrared Spectroscopy

Infrared spectroscopy (IR) has been used to study chain mobility in lipids and membranes. The band at 720 cm^{-1}, indicating trans CH_2 groups, decreases in intensity on going from crystal to liquid-crystal [35]. Infrared

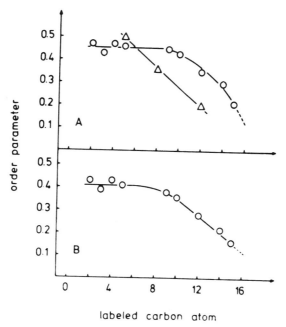

FIG. 8 Order parameter (S_{mol}) of diphosphatidyl PC bilayers as a function of the position of the labeled carbon atom. A. 41 °C; o——o, deuterium magnetic resonance (DMR) data; Δ——Δ, spin label data. B. 50 °C; o——o, DMR data. Reproduced from Seelig [164], with kind permission of the American Chemical Society.

spectroscopy studies are difficult because water bands interfere with the spectra. (IR studies on protein conformation in membranes are discussed later in this review.)

8. Enzymatic Probes

Considerations on the physical state of lipids are often extrapolated from studies of the temperature dependence of membrane-bound enzymes; that is, the properties of proteins are used as probes of the lipid environment. (Such studies will be described later.)

B. Lateral and Vertical Mobility of Lipids

In liquid-crystalline lipids, several techniques have shown that lateral motion of the individual molecules occurs very rapidly [28], with diffusion coefficients in the order of 10^{-8} cm^2/sec. Spin-labeling has been the most valuable technique in assessing lipid diffusion in bilayers, and three independent methods have given values around 10^{-8} cm^2/sec [106].

An indirect clue has been the demonstration that newly synthesized lipid molecules randomize rapidly in E. coli fatty acid auxotrophs [107]. Galla and Sackmann [93] have measured the diffusion of the lipid-soluble fluorophore pyrene, by formation of excited complexes between pyrene in the ground state and excited pyrene. The value found of D_{diff} for pyrene in pure lecithin at 50 °C was 1.4×10^{-7} cm^2/sec corresponding to 4×10^7 jumps per second, that is, a surface of 53,000 Å/sec. The diffusion rate of a molecule like pyrene buried in the hydrophobic region is expected to be higher than the intrinsic rate of amphipathic lipid molecules. Similar conclusions have been reached by Vanderkooi and Callis [108]. Lee et al. [109] have rationalized that lateral diffusion is the most plausible candidate for the intermolecular motion dominating the transverse relaxation time T_1 for PC vesicles. A self-diffusion coefficient for PC at 20 °C of 0.9×10^{-8} cm^2/sec was calculated, comparable with the values obtained by ESR.

While lateral mobility of lipid molecules appears a rather fast phenomenon, the jump of a lipid molecule from one to the other side of a bilayer (flipflop) occurs at a much lower rate [28, 110, 111]. The method used by Kornberg and McConnell [28] takes advantage of the impermeability of liposomes to ascorbate, which reduces nitroxides, thereby destroying their paramagnetic signal. Lipid vesicles are formed in a medium containing a spin-labeled phospholipid; ascorbate addition immediately destroys the nitroxides present in the external monolayer, while the rate of destruction of internal nitroxides depends on the rate of flipflop across the two monolayers (assuming no penetration by ascorbate). The exchange rate found was lower than 2×10^{-5} times per second.

IV. DISTRIBUTION OF LIPIDS IN BILAYERS AND MEMBRANES

There is increasing evidence that bilayers are asymmetric with respect to the lipids. Asymmetry has been detected in mixed phospholipid artificial vesicles obtained by sonication. Phosphatidyl ethanolamine (PE) is more heavily labeled by trinitrobenzenesulfonic acid (a membrane impermeable reagent that reacts with amino groups) when trapped inside the vesicles than when added externally [112]. The asymmetric distribution of PE and PC in mixed vesicles is lost at higher pH [113]. PE is zwitterionic and can be packed more tightly together at lower pH, and thus more molecules can populate the inner leaflet. An asymmetric distribution of cholesterol has been found in unsaturated PC vesicles by using the paramagnetic ion praseodymium to perturb the NMR signals of the choline groups in the different leaflet. In amounts up to 30%, cholesterol was found to distribute homogeneously, but over 30% it distributed to higher extents in the inner layer, while the less-packed unsaturated chains could be pushed aside [114]. This effect is not shown by saturated PC. Michaelson et al. [115], using paramagnetic ions to

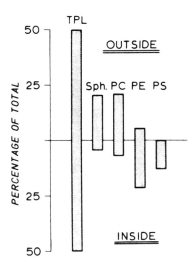

FIG. 9 Asymmetric distribution of phospholipids between inner and outer layer of the human erythrocyte membrane. Abbreviations: TPL, total phospholipids; Sph, sphingomyelin; PC, PE, PS have the usual meanings. Reproduced from Verkleij et al. [120], with kind permission of Elsevier Publishing Company.

quench NMR signals, found that vesicles containing equimolar quantities of PC and PG contain twice as much PG as PC in the outer surface, but within the surface the two classes were not segregated in patches. The reason for asymmetry has been attributed again in this case to the low radius of curvature and to the difference in charge, so that higher packing inside prevents PG insertion.

Evidence that PE, PC, and sphingomyelin are distributed asymmetrically in erythrocyte membranes has been found with nonpenetrating reagents [117-119], and by using phospholipases [120] and antibodies [121-124]. The study of Verkleij et al. [120] is worthy of detailed examination since it shows the sophistication reached in the combined use of phospholipases as probes of membrane structure. Phospholipase A_2 from Naja naja hydrolyzes 68% of PC of the intact human erythrocyte, and sphingomyelinase from S. aureus hydrolyzes up to 85% of total sphingomyelin. In intact cells treated first with phospholipase A and then with sphingomyelinase, about half the total phospholipids are degraded (mostly choline-containing phospholipids and some PE); treating erythrocyte ghosts, however, results in completed degradation.

The results suggest that most of the sphingomyelin and PC are located in the outer monolayer, while most PE and all PS are in the inner monolayer (Fig. 9). Phospholipase C from B. cereus does not attack intact cells but completely degrades glycerophospholipids from ghosts, with formation of

large diglyceride droplets. Phospholipase C can, however, degrade phospholipids in intact erythrocytes if they have been previously treated with sphingomyelinase; apparently, degradation of sphingomyelin exposes the lipids to
the action of phospholipase C.

Similar results have been obtained [125] by digesting sealed inside-out
vesicles from human erythrocytes with phospholipases A and C; virtually all
PE and PS and 30%–40% of PC and sphingomyelin were accessible, whereas
all phospholipids were accessible in unsealed ghosts.

In a study on the plasma membrane of Mycoplasma hominis, Rottem et al.
[126] have found that phospholipase C (B. cereus) fails to attack phospholipids
in intact cells or isolated membranes, but readily hydrolyzes the extracted
phospholipids dispersed in water, or membranes treated with proteolytic
enzymes. Moreover, binding of lysozyme to protein-depleted membranes
interferes with phospholipase C action. On the other hand, in membranes
reaggregated from solubilized subunits, there was a significant action of
phospholipase C, indicating that the reconstituted membranes differ from
the native membranes in organization. This study suggests that in M. hominis,
phospholipids are masked from enzymic attack by the presence of proteins.
The masking of phospholipase activity (both A and C) by basic proteins
ionically bound to the lipid bilayer has been shown by Lenaz et al. to occur
in phospholipid vesicles, but not in natural or reconstituted mitochondrial
membranes [127, 128]. The inefficiency of lysozyme in preventing phospholipid hydrolysis in membranes has been attributed to the patchy distribution
of neutral phosphoglycerides in mitochondrial membranes [127]. Studies on
fractionated mitochondria which have been treated with agents that degrade
phospholipids [129-132] suggest such a distribution in this inner membrane.

The asymmetry of lipids in a membrane may be accompanied by differences in fluidity in the two membrane halves. Rottem [133] suggests that in
A. laidlawii and M. hominis, the outer half of the membrane is more fluid
than the inner half, perhaps as a result of an asymmetry of proteins. A similar interpretation can be derived from findings of Wisnieski et al. [134].
Electron spin resonance analysis of plasma membranes reveals four characteristic temperatures for lateral phase separations, while only two such
temperatures appear in extracted lipids. The data could be interpreted in
terms of independent phase transitions for the inner monolayer (21 °C and
37 °C) and the outer monolayer (15 °C and 31 °C).

The reason for the differences in lipid composition found among the
inner and outer lipid monolayer in plasma membranes cannot be in the membrane curvature, as it is in artificial vesicles, but could be found in a bio-
synthetic difference. Renooij et al. [135] found that lecithin labeled by
incubation of radioactive fatty acids with human erythrocytes is found predominantly in the pool of lecithin localized in the inner monolayer, while
lecithin in the external monolayer may derive by exchange of the whole
molecule between plasma lipoproteins and the red-cell membrane [136].

V. PHOSPHOLIPID-CHOLESTEROL INTERACTION AS MODEL FOR PHOSPHOLIPID-PROTEIN INTERACTION

Phospholipid-cholesterol interactions may mimic phospholipid-protein interactions and give important indications of the forces involved. Moreover, cholesterol is a primary component of several membranes, which are strongly influenced by its presence. Cholesterol is an amphipathic molecule that becomes incorporated into hydrated phospholipid bilayers (or monolayers) up to a molar ratio of 1 cholesterol : 1 phospholipid [137]. Both components have their hydrophilic groups oriented towards water, while the hydrophobic sterol ring is in contact with fatty acid chains having at least ten carbon atoms [138].

Incorporating cholesterol was shown to condense lipid monolayers in the expanded state [5, 139, 140]. Condensation by cholesterol occurs in those lecithins that form expanded films, most strongly with those molecules that have a segment of saturated chain extending nine or more carbons from the carboxyl end [141]. Condensation by cholesterol results from increased packing efficiency. In compact films (saturated lecithins), cholesterol does not condense the bilayer, since the packing is already efficient. Also lecithins containing both polyunsaturated fatty acids (18:2, 18:3, etc.) give little condensation, since the chains have shorter saturated segments than C-9.

Spin-label, fluorescence, NMR, DSC, and other physical techniques in bilayer systems have confirmed the monolayer studies [21, 88, 137, 138, 142-149]. In addition, the following points have become apparent in bilayer studies. (1) Cholesterol decreases the motion of bilayer lipids only when the lipids are above the transition temperature. (2) Crystalline lipids on the other hand become more disordered by incorporation of cholesterol. (3) DSC shows that cholesterol abolishes the phase transition [5, 35, 137, 150, 151] (Fig. 10).

Dipalmitoyl lecithin has been studied by DSC and X-ray diffraction [152] over a wide range of temperatures. Adding cholesterol to the lecithin in water lowers the transition temperature slightly and decreases the heat absorbed at the transition, so that no transition at all is observed at 1 lecithin : 1 cholesterol. According to Oldfield and Chapman [150], the transition, although not detectable by DSC, is still present over a very wide temperature range and is noncooperative [153], contrary to the transition in absence of the sterol, which is a highly cooperative phenomenon.

In bilayers containing less than equimolar cholesterol, discrete regions of 1 : 1 complex separate out, leaving PC molecules at the boundaries of those regions for which cooperative motions are not possible, and clusters of free PC molecules in which the chains undergo cooperative motions and which freeze at the normal gel-liquid crystalline transition temperature (Fig. 11). Dipalmitoyl PC bilayers have completely homogeneous and saturated chains that below the transition are closely packed, owing to strong

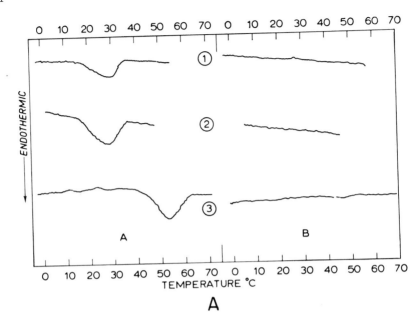

A

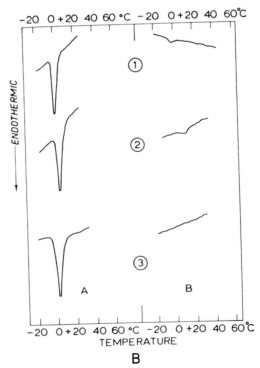

B

interaction between hydrocarbon chains and probably between headgroups also. Introducing cholesterol causes a forcing apart of the lipid molecules, with the sterol located between them, replacing some chain-chain interactions. The asymmetric shape of cholesterol relative to phospholipids results in a decreased lipid-lipid interaction, and increasing the cholesterol concentration gives rise to an increased amplitude of motion of the fatty acid chains [145, 154]. On the other hand, egg lecithin bilayers that are fluid at room temperature become oriented and rigidified by cholesterol, with decreased amplitude of the random walk angle of the fatty acid chains [145, 155]. Fluidization is accompanied by decrease of lateral separation and rigidization by increase of lateral separation, as evidenced by interacting spin label pairs as probes of lateral phase separation [144, 156]. The result of introducing cholesterol into a lipid bilayer is therefore to produce an intermediate phase (in the 1 : 1 complex) having less thermal motion above the transition of the phospholipid and more thermal motion below the transition [137].

As for the location and molecular relations of the interacting molecules, PMR has shown that the ten methylene groups in direct contact with the cholesterol nucleus are more immobilized than the groups at the end of the chains [157].

The PMR results are confirmed by ^{13}C magnetic resonance investigations [158] and are consistent with previous spin-label studies [159, 160] showing that near the methyl end of the chains the mobility is higher in presence of cholesterol than in the gel state, while the mobility is similar in the two states near the polar groups.

De Kruyff et al. [142] have studied the effect of the polar group of cholesterol on the lipid-cholesterol interaction. The 3β OH of sterol is essential for the condensing effect in monolayers and the reduction in energy content of thermal transition in liposomes. The hydration of the OH seems very important for the interaction, which is accompanied by an increase of bound water [142, 152].

When lipids in a bilayer are present in both fluid and solid phases, cholesterol preferentially interacts with liquid-crystalline lipids (at least at lower cholesterol concentrations [141, 142]) as visualized by freeze etching

---

FIG. 10 (Left) Effect of cholesterol on lipid phase transitions. A. Calorimetric scans of various lecithins: (1) rac-1-oleoyl-2-hexadecylglycero-3-phosphorylcholine; (2) rac-1-oleoyl-2-C-hexadecylpropanediol-3-phosphorylcholine, (3) 16:0/18:1 c-phosphorylcholine, (A) in the absence and (B) in the presence of 33.3 mole % cholesterol. B. Calorimetric scans of various pure lipids isolated from A. laidlawii: (1) PG (2) phosphoglycolipid, (3) diglucosyl diglyceride, (A) in the absence or (B) in the presence of 50 mole % cholesterol. Reproduced from De Kruyff et al. [138], with kind permission of Elsevier Publishing Company.

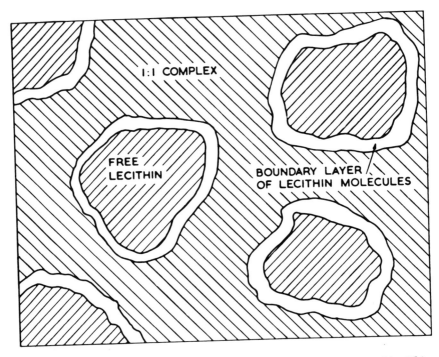

FIG. 11 Schematic representation of the structure of a mixed lecithin-cholesterol bilayer containing less than equimolar amounts of cholesterol. Reproduced from Phillips and Finer [143], with kind permission of Elsevier Publishing Company.

studies [38]. Thus cholesterol will not be randomly distributed in a membrane where phase separation may be present.

Cholesterol interaction with lipid bilayers has profound effects on permeability to ions and molecules. The permeability rates of anions, cations, and nonelectrolytes are considerably reduced in the presence of cholesterol [162]. This remarkable stabilizing effect is also present in natural membranes [163] and is related to the condensing effect. Further, cholesterol also inhibits the increase in cation transport induced by valinomycin [164] and by several proteins [165].

VI. EXTRACTION OF LIPIDS AND THEIR RECOMBINATION WITH PROTEINS

The possibility of removing lipids by solvent extraction or enzymatic attack without inducing gross morphological changes [166] has been used to

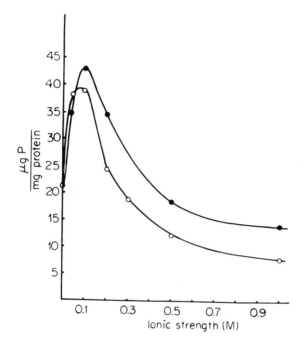

FIG. 12   Effect of salts on the binding of phospholipids to lipid-depleted mitochondria. ●——●, NaCl; o——o, NaSCN. Reproduced from Lenaz et al. [174], with kind permission of Academic Press.

examine the nature of the interaction between proteins and lipids and also the role lipids play in membrane function. For example, lipids can be added back to lipid-depleted mitochondria with recovery of succinoxidase activity [167], showing that the membrane recovers at least in part its native conformation. This interaction of phospholipids with lipid-depleted mitochondria is non-ionic and is stabilized primarily by hydrophobic bonds. The hydrophobic nature of the binding was first suggested for mitochondrial "structural protein" [168] with phospholipids [169]. "Structural protein" has been identified at least in part with denatured ATPase [170, 171], however. For this reason, studies with lipid-depleted mitochondria are more relevant to mitochondrial membrane structure. Lenaz et al. [172-175], by investigating the effect of ionic strength, pH, temperature, and solvents, have firmly established the hydrophobic nature of the interaction between phospholipids and lipid-depleted mitochondria. Similar conclusions were reached by Olivecrona and Oreland [176]. Hendler [177] raised the possibility that in recombination experiments, high salt may stimulate nonpolar binding at the same time that it depresses ionic interactions. The biphasic curve of the binding-vs-ionic strength (increase of binding at low ionic strength, and inhibition at high ionic strength) may be taken in favor of that hypothesis. The inhibition at high ionic strength, however, is stronger with chaotropic anions, which are known to break hydrophobic bonds by increasing the affinity of nonpolar residues for water [83]. Altogether, the characteristics of the binding suggest its hydrophobic nature (Fig. 12).

An initial ionic attraction is not a prerequisite for lipid to bind to lipid-depleted mitochondria. On the other hand, Zwaal and Van Deenen [178, 179], in studying the recombination of erythrocyte membrane proteins solubilized in water after butanol extraction with membrane lipids, have found that recombination of lipids does not occur at physiological pH or in presence of 0.2 M NaCl. Once the complex is formed, however, changes in pH or increased ionic strength do not split the complex. In this case, the association of proteins and lipids requires previous electrostatic interaction, which is then stabilized by hydrophobic bonds, as also indicated by immobilization of the methylene groups of the lipids measured by NMR [180]. Similarly, the recombination of human erythrocyte apoprotein with lipids at the air–water interface has both ionic and hydrophobic components [181].

It seems reasonable to correlate the need for an initial ionic attraction with the water solubility of the protein used [182]. Solubilized erythrocyte proteins must have a different conformation in comparison with the original membranes. The transition from a membranous state to a water–soluble one and vice versa must necessarily involve a conformational change of the molecule, with exposure of polar groups to the exterior. On the other hand, when membranes are rendered lipid-deficient by acetone extraction or phospholipase digestion, they remain in an insoluble form, resembling the original membrane [166], and thus with exposed hydrophobic residues, so that interaction with added phospholipids will be directly hydrophobic without any need for a previous ionic attraction (Fig. 13).

This latter case describes the recombination of proteins and lipids dissolved in organic solvents like 2–chloroethanol. Zahler and Weibel [183] have recombined 2–chloroethanol-dissolved erythrocyte lipids and proteins by dialysis against aqueous buffers. Ionic strength had no effect on their reconstitution, showing that the recombination is hydrophobic as expected from the previous exposure to a hydrophobic medium, which would not be expected to alter the specific membrane conformation. Similar results were obtained by Kramer et al. [184], who in addition observed a selectivity of membrane proteins for binding different lipids.

Schubert et al. [185] reported that recombination of erythrocyte proteins, extracted with acetic acid, was independent of the ionic environment. According to Juliano [186], this anomalous effect, contrasting with the results of Zwaal and Van Deenen, must be due to the maintenance of the membrane conformation after acetic acid treatment. The incorporation into black lipid membranes of erythrocyte proteins, extracted by different techniques, has been attempted by several investigators [187–189]. Adding a strongly bound

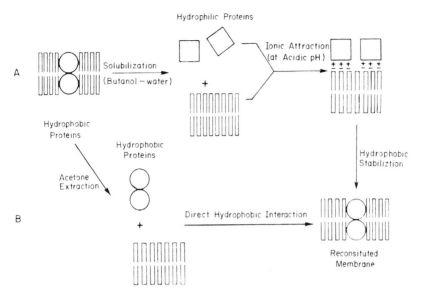

FIG. 13 Two different types of lipid-protein interactions. A. Membranes solubilized with butanol-water. The water-soluble proteins are reconstituted with phospholipids at acidic pH [178]. B. Membranes delipidated by means of acetone or by phospholipase digestion.

fraction (containing the sialoglycoprotein) elicits a 10^3-fold increase in electrical conductivity of oxidized cholesterol membranes.

Studies with several membranes have shown that solubilization by means of certain detergents (e.g. deoxycholate) may result in lipid extraction from the solubilized proteins (see Chap. 1). This effect has been the basis for the work of reconstitution of mitochondrial membranes in the laboratory of D. E. Green [190]. Dialyzing depolymerized "units" in the presence of lipids removes detergent and allows the "units" to realign spontaneously, and reforming vesicular membranes. Studies along this line were the basis for the suggestion [191] that the process of membrane assembly consists in the bidimensional association of lipoprotein "repeating units" along a plane, with phospholipids functioning to provide a more extensive hydrophilic surface and thus to prevent polymerization in the third dimension. This concept appears still valid today, although in certain cases the membrane structure may appear to be changed by the solubilization-reconstitution treatment, as recognized by irreversible changes of certain membrane properties, for example in SDS-solubilized membranes of A. laidlawii [192] and in SDS-solubilized membranes of M. lysodeikticus [193].

Extraction procedures show that it is often difficult to extract a fraction of membrane lipids with the usual solvent mixtures, drastic procedures being called for. This difficulty is not related to the nature of the lipid material, and seems to depend on the way they are bound in the membrane.

Moreover, the "tightly bound" lipids do not correspond quantitatively to the lipids that are strongly immobilized as detected by spin-label experiments. The tightly bound cardiolipin found in cytochrome oxidase membranes by Awasthi et al. [194] would account, from Vanderkooi's calculations [195] for about 25% of the boundary lipids.

The problem of tightly bound lipids is still unclear in their relation to membrane structure. Following the pioneering studies of Parpart and Ballentine [196], Roelofsen et al. [197] confirmed that ether removes only a specific portion of the lipids from lyophilized erythrocyte membranes. They concluded that since the differential extraction is not due to specific solubility of different lipid classes in the organic solvent, different types of interactions have to be present with the membrane proteins. All classes of phospholipids are present in both loosely and tightly bound lipids, but quantitatively PE prevails in the loosely bound fraction. Similar differential extractability was found in mitochondria [198, 199]. Lenaz et al. [199] also found that in membranes depleted of extrinsic proteins, the loosely bound phospholipids contain mainly PE.

The need of solvents containing ionic components (ammonia) to extract the tightly bound lipids suggests that both ionic and hydrophobic interactions may be involved in their linkage to proteins. The more tightly bound lipids may be those forming ion pairs with protein-charged groups as discussed by Gitler and Montal [200, 201].

It is also possible that the nonpolar moieties of lipids, more closely associated with protein, may interdigitate with nonpolar amino acid residues, as described in the model by Benson [202], very popular some years ago. Such a model could be valid on a limited scale for some of the most tightly bound lipids.

VII. THE ROLE OF LIPIDS IN MEMBRANE FUNCTIONS

Lipids represent a hydrophobic environment for intrinsic membrane proteins. According to Vanderkooi [203], a membrane can be viewed as a concentrated solution of lipids and proteins in two dimensions. By analogy with bulk tridimensional solutions, they may be in either a liquid or a solid state. For solutions with a low-to-moderate viscosity, the membrane will behave as a two-dimensional fluid. For such solutions, a certain time-average number of protein-protein contacts will always exist but the identity of the individual contacts will be continuously changing in a liquidlike manner. Cross-linking reagents such as glutaraldehyde will freeze the protein distribution by producing permanent bonds. Vanderkooi [195] has examined the thermodynamics of two-dimensional solutions in order to derive simple rules concerning the miscibility of proteins and lipids.

Taking the assumption that lipids represent a medium for intrinsic proteins, a unifying theory can be proposed for the role of lipids in the function of membrane proteins. It has been known for a long time that lipids are required for activity for many membrane-bound enzymes [191] but they are also involved in protein metabolism and amino acid transport [204]. A self-proposing role of lipids in membrane-linked activities is their being a medium with well-defined characteristics (low polarity and dielectric constant, high viscosity) suitable for inducing or stabilizing an optimal conformation in the hydrophobic proteins associated with membrane activities. The role of lipids, however, is quite complex and several other functions have been advanced for lipids in membranes. A role in stabilizing the conformation of membrane proteins has not been studied extensively.

A. Lipid Requirements for Intrinsic Membrane Enzymes

The involvement of lipids in the function of membrane enzymes was first demonstrated when it was shown that rebinding phospholipids to solvent-extracted mitochondria leads to reactivation of respiratory activity [167]. Subsequently it was demonstrated that phospholipids are required for each segment of the respiratory chain both in intact mitochondria and in purified systems [205, 206] and for a variety of enzymic activities of several other membranes [cf. 30, 182, 207, 208].

Certain enzymes appear to have an absolute requirement or at least a preference for certain phospholipid classes. The ($Na^+ + K^+$) ATPase appears to require PS or other negatively charged phospholipids [209]. An example of absolute specificity (lecithin) is the mitochondrial β-hydroxybutyrate dehydrogenase [210]. In contrast, PE but not lecithin is effective in reactivating the glucose-6-phosphatase activity lost on phospholipase C digestion [211].

There is very little specificity of phospholipid classes in restoration of respiratory activity in lipid-depleted mitochondria [167]. Different phospholipid fractions are active, although cardiolipin is effective at lower concentrations than lecithin. Tightly bound cardiolipin, however, seems specific in cytochrome oxidase activity [194]. The problem of lipid specificity in mitochondrial function has been pursued by Racker in his experiments on reconstituting isolated segments of the respiratory chain and oxidative phosphorylation. For example, the third site of oxidative phosphorylation was reconstituted by combining phospholipids, cytochrome oxidase, cytochrome c, and preparations of oligomycin-sensitive ATPase. After the cholate used to solubilize the system was removed by dialysis, vesicles were formed from which external cytochrome c was removed. In this system, PC and PE together provided a phospholipid mixture for maximal activity, as long as unsaturated fatty acids were present [212, 213].

In vesicles catalyzing ^{32}Pi-ATP exchange and ATP-driven proton translocation and free of electron-transfer carriers, PC and PE were required in
the ratio 4 PE:1 PC for optimal activity. When these substances were present
in equimolar amounts, the rate was accelerated by small amounts of cardiolipin. Unsaturated fatty acids were required absolutely for reconstituted
activity [214]. Similarly, the ability to phosphorylate ADP during oxidation
of NADH by Q_1 was restored to the NADH-CoQ reductase complex by combining the latter with a hydrophobic protein and phospholipids [215]. Here
there was an absolute requirement for PE and a partial requirement for PC
(with 4 : 1 optimal ratio); in the presence of low cardiolipin (0.05%–1.5%),
the optimal ratio becomes 1 PE : 1 PC.

Stimulation of mitochondrial ATPase by PC was studied in a lipid-free
preparation from beef-heart mitochondria obtained by cholate extraction
[216]. The low stimulatory activity of PC was increased either by introducing
negative amphipathic substances into the zwitterionic liposomes or by adding
Cl$^-$ to the incubation medium. Liposomes of acidic phospholipids or PC containing anionic phospholipids prevented the (ATP + Mg^{2+})-induced decrease
of ATPase activity in submitochondrial particles containing the ATPase inhibitor subunit. Acidic phospholipids (not PC) prevented the inhibition of soluble
or particulate ATPase by purified ATPase inhibitor.

From the examples considered, it seems that although the extent of
specificity may be different, with a few exceptions those phospholipids bearing
a net negative charge are more efficient in restoring membrane activities.

There may be several reasons at once why lipids are required for membrane enzyme activities. The complex situation described above concerning
the specificity of the required lipids suggests that each system under study
might be unique in its particular properties.

B. Function of Lipids as a Binding Site for Extrinsic Enzymes

Binding to a membrane can modify enzyme activity by changing the enzyme
microenvironment [217, 218]. In certain instances, phospholipids have been
found to determine the binding of enzymes to membranes. Phospholipid
digestion with phospholipase A releases NADH dehydrogenase [219] and
β-hydroxybutyrate dehydrogenase [220] from mitochondrial membranes.
Release of NADH dehydrogenase has been correlated with hydrolysis of
cardiolipin because Crotalus adamanteus phospholipase, which is inert
towards cardiolipin, does not release the enzyme under conditions in which
Naja naja phospholipase is successful. The release of glutamic-aspartic
transaminase and glutamate dehydrogenase from rat-liver mitochondria
incubated at 30 °C is inhibited by purified phospholipids, which protect the
membrane from the effect of endogenous phospholipase [221]. These observations suggest that the released enzymes are bound to phospholipids in the
intact membranes.

Certain enzymes have been found to require lipids when in soluble form although they are lipid–dependent when bound to the native membrane; such is the case for brain hexokinase [222], pyruvate dehydrogenase, and α–keto-glutarate dehydrogenase complexes [191].

C. Latency and Compartmentation

Compartmentation is one important aspect of cellular function imposed by the hydrophobic properties of lipids. The importance of compartmentation is observed at many levels of cellular organization and function. Secretory processes of proteins from exocrine and endocrine glands involve membrane fusion phenomena [223–225].

Activation of lysosomal enzymes is a primary aspect of compartmentation. Treatments leading to "activation" of these enzymes include mechanical breakage, or reaction with detergents, phospholipases, and proteases [225]. Studies in vitro on the conditions inducing release of latent enzymes involve formation of artificial lipid vesicles containing included enzymes [e.g., 226]. Activation of many membrane enzymes by detergents or phospholipases may involve "opening" phenomena with loss of compartmentation.

Of course, transport phenomena require lipids as the hydrophobic determinants of the membrane continuity. Lipids appear essential for transport; the net charge of the membrane, the phospholipid–to–sterol ratio, and the nature of the component fatty acids have large effects on ion transport [227]. In addition, lipids are required for enzymic systems that are essential parts of transport systems.

Oxidative phosphorylation in mitochondria and photophosphorylation in chloroplasts and photosynthetic bacteria appear to involve proton translocation across the energy–conserving membranes [228]. The energy–conserving process requires a proton–impermeable membrane and the Δ pH + $\Delta\psi$ gradient is physiologically discharged by the ATP-synthesizing ATPase. Phospholipids are impermeable to protons as well as to cations. Uncoupling agents of phosphorylation are weak acids capable of traversing the membrane in undissociated form, thereby discharging protons and short–circuiting the electrochemical gradient established by the proton–translocating respiratory or photosynthetic chains. According to this view, both respiratory complexes and ATPase are H^+–conducting channels inserted in the phospholipid bilayer (Fig. 14).

The success Racker and his coworkers obtained in reconstituting oxidative phosphorylation is related to formation of closed impermeable vesicles that do not allow free equilibration of H^+. The sidedness, or directionality, of transport is linked to correct disposition of the proton carriers in the membrane. Let us take the example of reconstitution of the third coupling site in cytochrome oxidase vesicles [212] (Fig. 15). Recombination of cytochrome oxidase with lipid bilayers is expected to be random—in other words, is

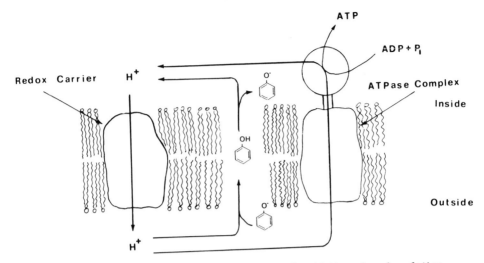

FIG. 14 Schematic view of mitochondrial oxidative phosphorylation according to the chemio-osmotic hypothesis. The proton pressure established outside the inner mitochondrial membrane by electron transport reverses a proton-transporting asymmetric ATPase, thus driving ATP synthesis. Uncoupling is depicted as short-circuiting of protons through lipophilic weak acids (phenols), to which the membrane is permeable in the undissociated form.

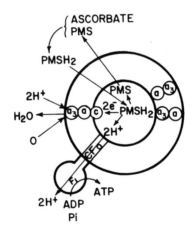

SMP MODEL

FIG. 15 Reconstitution of the third site of oxidative phosphorylation. Electron transfer in the SMP (submitochondrial particle) model occurs only from reduced phenazine methosulfate ($PMSH_2$) inside the vesicles to oxygen outside, through the sequence of cytochromes c, a, and a_3 in that order. At the same time, hydrogen ions are transferred through the ATPase membrane factor (here called CF_0) to F_1, and ATP is synthesized from ADP and Pi. Reproduced from Racker [212], with kind permission of Academic Press.

expected not to involve a uniform directionality of the proton-translocating channel. Adding cytochrome c (the electron-donating substrate) to only one side, however, imposes vectoriality to the otherwise random system, so that protons are translocated only into the medium on the side at which cytochrome c is bound. Only in this way is a proton gradient established. This gradient can be discharged by the H^+-translocating ATPase, and ATP synthesis is achieved.

Light-driven phosphorylation has been reconstituted from a liposome system containing only bacteriorhodopsin and ATPase [229]. Light induces proton translocation across the reconstituted lipid vesicle through bacteriorhodopsin, and ATPase discharges the gradient and synthesizes ATP.

For these phenomena, lipids are apparently required as a medium separating two different aqueous media and imposing vectoriality to specific proton transport systems. It is likely that the lipids involved in these less specific functions are "free bilayer" lipids not in direct contact with membrane proteins.

D. Solvent Action of Lipids

One role of lipids in certain membrane functions may be to provide a suitable environment for processes requiring nonpolar media.

Coenzyme Q, or ubiquinone [230], is a lipid-soluble molecule involved in electron transport between the flavoprotein region and cytochrome b in the mitochondrial respiratory chain. The pool function of CoQ in electron transport has been suggested by Green [231] and confirmed by Kröger and Klingenberg [232]. In view of its long isoprene chain, CoQ must be localized in the lipid phase and move back and forth to transfer electrons between carriers that are part of fixed lipoprotein complexes within the membrane [233].

Enzymes involved in lipid metabolism also usually have a phospholipid requirement [30, 182]. In this case, lipids may be required for an appropriate binding area for hydrophobic substrates. For this effect, enzymes do not appear to require a bilayer structure; a micellar binding interface is adequate, as proved for C_{55}-isoprenoid alcohol phosphokinase [234].

Rothfield [235-238] has studied the interaction of UDP-glucose:lipopolysaccharide glycosyl transferase and UDP-galactose:lipopolysaccharide α,3-galactosyltransferase with phospholipids and found an absolute lipid requirement for glycosyl transfer to lipopolysaccharide in the presence of the purified enzymes. The main function of phospholipids is to interact with the lipopolysaccharide substrate, and the transferase molecules are intercalated into the basic lipid-lipopolysaccharide framework. This model was also supported by the reconstitution of the complex in monolayers possessing full activity [239, 240]. In this well-characterized system, the role of lipids seems mostly linked to the alignment of the substrate molecules, but probably involves also penetration of the phospholipid-substrate complex by the enzyme (Fig. 16).

Dawson [241] has examined the specificity and role of phospholipids in enzymes involved in phospholipid metabolism. Among the physical factors

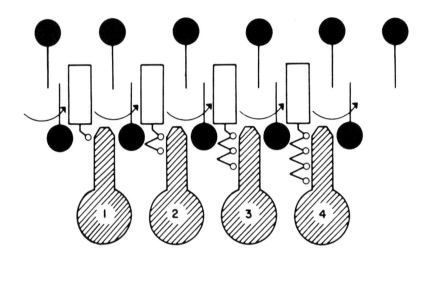

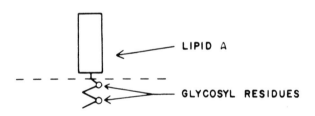

FIG. 16 Model of localization of glycosyl transferases in the membrane.
The enzymes are located adjacent to each other and lipopolysaccharides
(rectangles) are free to migrate laterally along the chain of enzymes. Alternatively, the enzymes are also free to migrate. Reproduced from Rothfield
and Hinckley [238], with kind permission of North-Holland Publishing Company

affecting enzymatic reactions is the physical form of lipids participating in
the reactions (as substrates and activators at the same time). The hydrophobicity of the substrate could enhance lipase activity by three factors:
unfolding of the enzyme with exposure of the active site, hydrophobic binding
of substrate to the active site, and shielding of hydrophilic esters by organized
water against the attack of a weakly nucleophilic enzyme. Pieterson et al.
[242] have proposed a kinetic model describing the action of soluble enzymes
(such as pancreatic phospholipase A_2) at interfaces, in terms of two successive equilibria: (1) a rate-limiting reversible penetration by the enzyme of

the interface, and (2) formation of the Michaelis complex. Phospholipase A_2 contains a hydrophobic region (penetration site) functionally different from the active site. It is also thought that during penetration the protein undergoes a conformational change, in which the optimal alignment of the active site is reached [243]. The pancreatic phospholipase A_2 zymogen has the active site but lacks the penetration site, since it is unable to attack phospholipids in micellar form but hydrolyzes only monomeric phospholipids. The hydrolysis is high only near the transition temperature [244]. Enhanced lateral compressibility when liquid and solid phases coexist will induce better insertion of the hydrophobic penetration site. On the other hand, Wells [245], using Crotalus adamanteus phospholipase A_2, has found no evidence of hydrophobic interaction, and the role of lipids in this case could be that such an interface provides many more productive collisions than the surface of a monomer tumbling in solution.

Other factors affecting action of lipid-specific enzymes [246] are the ratio between substrate mass and the area of interface available for enzymic attack, the extent of molecular packing, solvent addition (by diluting the polar groups), and the electrostatic field (perhaps affecting adsorption and penetration of the enzymes).

E. Molecularization and Membrane Formation

Green and Tzagoloff [191] have suggested that membrane formation consists of bidimensional association of lipoprotein "subunits" along a plane, and

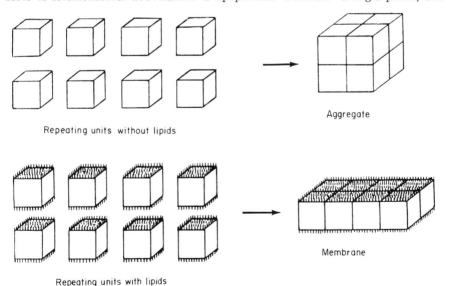

Aggregate

Repeating units without lipids

Membrane

Repeating units with lipids

FIG. 17 Role of lipids in membrane formation, after Green and Tzagoloff [191].

that the function of phospholipids is to provide a hydrophilic surface preventing polymerization in the third dimension (Fig. 17).

Reassembly of disaggregated subunits gives rise to vesicles resembling the original membrane when lipids are present [190]. However, changes in the nature of the bonds stabilizing the membrane may occur, as evidenced by physical means [192, 193] and by the fact that enzymic activities are only partly restored. According to Green and Tzagoloff [190], the structural role of lipids in membrane formation may also explain the lipid dependence of several enzyme systems. Aggregation as opposed to molecularization (i.e., formation of bidimensional membranes) will not allow a functional contact of reactive groups and substrates. Soluble enzymes are spontaneously "molecularized" in water and are not lipid-dependent. In the case of water-insoluble enzymes, molecularization represents restriction of polymerization only along a plane; that is membrane formation.

F. Role of Lipids in Maintaining the Active Conformation of Membrane Enzymes

The processes described above cannot explain alone the lipid dependence of certain enzyme systems. For example, the observation that lipid-depleted mitochondria conserve a bidimensional appearance of electron microscopy [166] but are devoid of respiratory activity is not fully compatible with some of the previous interpretations. One could envisage, however, that lipids impose a finer level of organization, which functions to direct the precise contact between individual proteins in multiprotein complexes to assure that multistep catalysis occurs in a concerted way. In other words, the lipid-free enzymes are not in the proper environmental conditions.

But the most stimulating idea is that phospholipids may be involved as regulators of enzymic activities by inducing the proper conformation in the enzymic proteins. It is reasonable that enzymes linked to biomembranes or having penetrating regions assume their optimal conformation when the highest number of hydrophobic residues are situated on the exterior of the protein molecule in contact with the nonpolar hydrocarbon regions of the lipids.

Evidence for conformational changes induced by lipids on proteins arises from numerous studies, most of which involve kinetics of membrane-linked enzymes. It is reasonable that in many cases kinetic changes should be the result of protein conformational changes. This subject has been reviewed recently in detail [29, 247] and will be summarized here only in its salient features. Examples are reported in Table 3.

Affinities for substrates or inhibitors either increase or decrease on solubilization of membrane enzymes. In a model study [261], rabbit muscle lactate dehydrogenase was covalently bound to glass beads. The refolded covalently bound subunits were capable of enzymic activity and recombination with native subunits. The bound enzyme exhibited an increase in K_M for NADH and a decrease for pyruvate; the latter effect may only reflect a conformational change induced by the matrix environment. Also K_D for NAD decreased, suggesting a structural change resulting in more favorable binding. Dodd [262] found that glutamate and malate dehydrogenases, considered soluble mitochondrial matrix enzymes, bind very strongly to phospholipid bilayers by both ionic and hydrophobic interactions. Binding of glutamate dehydrogenase to cardiolipin or PS is accompanied by strong inhibition of activity; the interaction and inhibition are counteracted by high ionic strength. Dodd postulated that the enzyme is physiologically bound to the inner membrane in an inactive form, and that an intramitochondrial increase of NH_4^+ would activate glutamate formation by detaching the enzyme as a result of loosening ionic interactions. As NH_4^+ is used up in the reaction

$$\alpha\text{-ketoglutarate} + NH_4^+ + NADH + H^+ \rightarrow \text{glutamate} + NAD^+ + H_2O$$

the ionic strength comes back to normal, and the enzyme rebinds to the membrane in the inactive form.

Removing membrane lipids usually results in loss or decrease of enzymic activities; the inactivation is often a consequence of a decrease in V_{max}. In fact, in many examples, the K_M for substrate also decreases, indicating that a decreased affinity of the enzyme for its substrate is not the reason for loss of activity. A clue to the nature of this effect comes from a study of Hégyvary [260] on the effect of organic solvents on $(Na^+ + K^+)$-ATPase. Inhibition by alcohols was found to be uncompetitive with respect to ATP. In the presence of these solvents, the apparent affinity of the enzyme increased for Na^+ and ATP and decreased for K^+. By pulse-labeling, it was shown that organic solvents enhance the interaction of ATP with the enzyme prior to phosphorylation, both in the presence and in the absence of K^+. On the other hand, they decrease the rate of dephosphorylation of phosphoenzyme in the presence of K^+. The uncompetitive type of inhibition (decrease of both V_{max} and K_M simultaneously) indicates an increased stability of the enzyme-substrate Michaelis complex, with decreased k_3, that is decreased product formation. On the other hand, in Electrophorus electroplax, Goldman and Albers [263] found that PE removal increases the stability of the Mg^{2+}-enzyme complex, while PS is required for the formation of the phosphorylated intermediate as well as for its dephosphorylation.

In Ca^{2+} ATPase of sarcoplasmic reticulum, phospholipids are not required for formation of phosphoenzyme intermediate; they are necessary, however, for subsequent hydrolysis of the phosphorylated intermediate [264, 265].

It is of interest that phospholipase A_2 treatment of submitochondrial particles also induces an uncompetitive inhibition, with decrease of both V_{max} and K_M for ATP [Lenaz and coworkers, unpublished] (Fig. 18). This suggests that a phosphorylated intermediate of the ATPase reaction is more stable, with decrease of both k_3 and k_2 in the following reaction:

$$ATP + E \underset{k_2}{\overset{k_1}{\rightleftharpoons}} E\text{-}P \longrightarrow E + Pi$$

TABLE 3

Effect of Lipids on the K_M of Membrane-Bound Enzymes

Treatment	Enzyme	K_M	Reference
Solubilization (detergent)	Glucose-6-phosphatase	Decreased	248
	Glucose-6-phosphatase, glucose-inhibited	Increased	249
	Hexokinase (brain)	Increased	250
	Acetylcholinesterase	Decreased	251
Delipidation	Pyruvate oxidase	Increased	252, 253
	Glucose-6-phosphatase	Decreased	254
	UDP-glucuronyl transferase	Decreased	255
	Succinate-cyt. c reductase	Decreased	256
	Cytochrome oxidase	Decreased	257
	Mitochondrial ATPase	Decreased	Lenaz (unpublished)
	Mitochondrial ATPase (isolated enzyme)	Increased	258
Solvents	Na-K ATPase	Unaffected	259
	Na-K ATPase	Decreased	260
	Mitochondrial ATPase	Decreased	29

Note: Selected examples only.

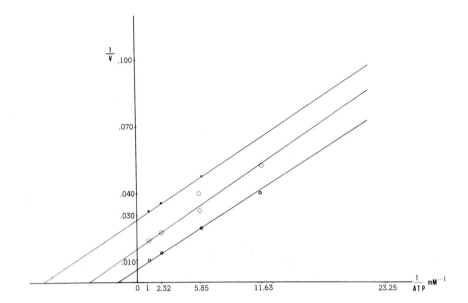

FIG. 18 Double reciprocal plot of ATPase activity: effect of phospholipase A_2 (Naja naja). o——o, no addition; ⊖——⊖, + phospholipase A_2 (5-min incubation); ●——●, + phospholipase A_2 (10-min incubation).

In isolated oligomycin-sensitive ATPase, however, Swanljung et al. [258] found that phospholipid reactivation was accompanied by decrease of K_M.

Lenaz et al. [29] have found that the effect of several solvents and anesthetics on mitochondrial ATPase is an uncompetitive inhibition with respect to ATP, in accord with the phospholipase data.

Delipidation also decreases the K_M of succinate-cytochrome c reductase for succinate and PMS [256] and the K_M of cytochrome oxidase for cytochrome c [257]. In a few cases, delipidation was found to increase the K_M, as in the case of pyruvate oxidase [252, 253].

A role of lipids is also apparent in hormone action and adenyl cyclase mediation of hormone activity [266]; specific phospholipids elicit specific hormonal responses on adenyl cyclase activity [267] but hormone binding is generally not affected by delipidation, suggesting that lipids are required to transmit a signal from the hormone receptor to the cyclase catalytic site on the other side of the membrane.

For complex activities like electron transport and the activity of ATPase in mitochondria and other membranes, multiple subunits combine to determine the overall activity.

Mitochondrial ATPase [268-270] is a very complex enzyme (Fig. 19), which in situ is able to catalyze ATP synthesis coupled with a flow of protons

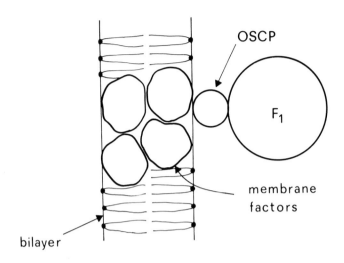

FIG. 19 Schematic view of the mitochondrial ATPase.

from the outer medium (where they have been extruded by electron transfer) to the matrix [228]. A catalytic unit, composed of five types of extrinsic subunits, contains the active site for ATP hydrolysis. This complex has been isolated as a water-soluble protein by Pullman et al. [271] and is identical with the factor F_1, that restores oxidative phosphorylation in deficient submitochondrial particles. In addition, the membrane-bound ATPase contains a protein called oligomycin-sensitivity-conferring protein (OSCP) [272], which links F_1 and the membrane and for this reason is needed to confer oligomycin sensitivity. The true component that confers oligomycin sensitivity to ATPase and may constitute the H^+ channel [273] is a "membrane factor" [274], consisting of four proteins, which in yeast are products of mitochondrial protein synthesis and are very hydrophobic. Finally, a soluble ATPase inhibitor peptide inhibits ATPase activity during oxidative phosphorylation [275]. When mitochondrial protein synthesis is inhibited, cytoplasmic products of ATPase (F_1 and OSCP) are still synthesized, but they are not integrated into the membrane; thus, the overall ATPase activity is modulated by the membrane [274]. Phospholipids are required for ATPase activity in membranes and in the isolated oligomycin-sensitive complex [258, 276, 277], but not in F_1. The role of phospholipids may be to maintain the correct conformation of F_1 (through the membrane factors) and its correct binding to the membrane. Acidic phospholipids remove the inhbition of particulate ATPase by the natural ATPase inhibitor [276]. The inhibition of ATPase by oligomycin or DCCD requires the presence of the "membrane factor" that contains the inhibitor binding site in one of its component proteins [278, 279]; phospholipids are required for inhibition to occur [280].

The change of ATPase properties in the soluble and bound form was first recognized by Racker [281], and called allotopy. Allotopy may be a general property of membrane-bound enzymic complexes.

Solvents have been found to affect the allotopic properties of membrane-bound enzymes. Alcohols make the ATPase oligomycin and DCCD insensitive with an efficacy depending on alcohol hydrophobicity [29, 282]. The concentration of n-butanol required for this effect corresponds to that which disrupts protein-lipid interactions as probed by spin labels [29, 283]. The ATPase is not detached from the membrane in these experiments, indicating that only dislocation of F_1 from the membrane factors has occurred. Ether induces similar changes [90, 282, 284]. Azzi et al. [285] have shown that ether abolishes the spin-spin interaction of Mn-ATP with a paramagnetic DCCD analog, demonstrating that the distance of the ATP site in F_1 from the DCCD-binding protein increases after ether treatment from 20 Å to > 35 Å. Also, general anesthetics [29] abolish oligomycin sensitivity. Since the effects run parallel to changes in lipid fluidity and disruption of lipid-protein interactions, it is tempting to relate the two phenomena, on the basis that allotopic properties of mitochondrial ATPase depend on membrane lipids. The translation of the specific oligomycin or DCCD sensitivity from the membrane factors into a conformational change of the catalytic unit may be impaired when the lipid environment of the membrane factors is modified by the solvents.

Changes in the allosteric behavior of certain membrane-bound enzymes were found in rats fed fat-deficient diets or diets having different lipid compositions [e.g., 286-288]. In rats fed a fat-free diet the allosteric kinetics for fluoride inhibition of ATPase changed from Hill coefficients n = -2 to n = -1, and a relation was found with a change of the double bond index-saturation ratio, indicative of fluidity. It appears that membrane fluidity is a physiological regulator of the allosteric behavior of membrane enzymes, indicating conformational differences in the different situations. Thus for membrane-bound Ca^{2+} ATPase from E. Coli, the cooperativity of this enzyme at 36 °C is enhanced, while that at 19 °C is lowered, in comparison with these allosteric properties of the soluble enzymes [289].

The effects of loading membranes with cholesterol in vitro are also consistent with a direct relation between membrane fluidity and the allosteric behavior of certain enzymes [290].

It has been suggested that membrane fluidity mediates the action of hormones. Insulin and cortisol affect the Hill coefficients of rat-erythrocyte acetylcholinesterase and (Na^+-K^+) ATPase in opposite ways, indicating that insulin decreases and cortisol enhances membrane fluidity [291].

In the case of enzymes with only a weak interaction with membranes, variations of the allosteric behavior (Hill plots) and not Arrhenius plots are needed to evaluate lipid-induced conformational changes [292, 293]. The reason may be a thermodynamic one, since changes of the order of 0.7-0.8 Kcal/mole are needed to detect a change in position of the break in an Arrhenius plot [294].

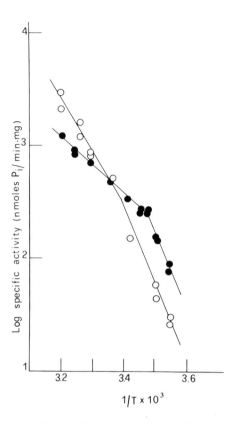

FIG. 20 Arrhenius plot of ATPase activity in beef-heart mitochondria.
●——●, no addition; o——o, + Triton X-100, 2.5 mg/ml.

Anomalies in the temperature dependence of membrane activities have
been related to transitions in the physical state of membrane lipids [29, 247,
295, 296]. Arrhenius plots of soluble enzymes generally show straight lines
with constant activation energies over a wide range of temperatures. In contrast, for membrane-bound enzymes the plots show sharp breaks or discontinuities with different activation energies, E_A being higher below the
discontinuity (Fig. 20).

The interpretation of the discontinuities has been discussed by Kumamoto
et al. [297]. Two independent processes having different E_A are required to
produce a discontinuity, with the process having the higher E_A operating
exclusively at temperatures below the discontinuity. It has been assumed
that the system undergoes a phase change at the break temperature, and that
in turn, the perturbation associated with such change in the enzyme environment induces a conformational change in the protein, so that the conformation

with higher E_A exists below the critical temperature. A direct correlation between the inflection point in an Arrhenius plot and a conformational change was found by Massey et al. [298] for a soluble enzyme. No such correlation is as yet available for membrane-bound enzymes.

The phase change is usually ascribed to the lipid environment, and breaks in Arrhenius plots of membrane enzymes usually coincide with critical temperatures associated with the phase transitions in lipids. Some typical examples and references are reported in Table 4; a more extensive literature is reported in other reviews [cf. e.g. 29]. Raison and McMurchie [64] found that the lipid components of mitochondrial membranes show abrupt changes in molecular ordering at two temperatures with concomitant changes in activation energy for succinate oxidation (Fig. 21). The two breaks were correlated with the onset and completion of lateral phase separation [cf. 307, 308]. In one study, however, no such correspondence was found [309]:

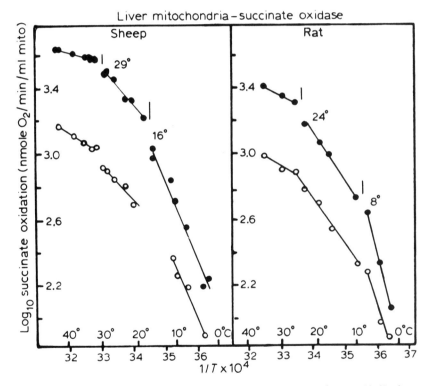

FIG. 21 Two breaks in Arrhenius plots of succinoxidase activity in sheep-liver and rat-liver mitochondria. ●——●, state III respiration; o——o, state IV respiration. Reproduced from Raison and McMurchie [64], with kind permission of Elsevier Publishing Company.

TABLE 4

Some Examples of Discontinuities in Arrhenius Plots of Membrane-Bound Enzymes

Source	Function	Treatment	Temperature (°C)		Reference
Mitochondria	Energy-linked reactions involving adenine nucleotides		17.5	27.5	299
	Energy-linked reactions not involving adenine nucleotides		12.5	27.5	299
Mitochondria (rat liver)	Succinate oxidation		24	8	64
Mitochondria (sheep liver)	Succinate oxidation		29	16	64
Mitochondria (beef heart)	ATPase		16		300
	Succinate oxidation		26		300
	Cytochrome oxidase		26		296
	β-hydroxybutyrate dehydrogenase		18.5		300
Kidney	(Na–K) ATPase (isolated, delipidated)	+ Dimyristoyl PG	20		301
		+ Dipalmitoyl PG	31.4		
		+ Distearoyl PG	44.3		
		+ Dioleyl PG	None		
Erythrocytes	(Na–K) ATPase		20		Lenaz, Curatola (unpublished)
Mycoplasma mycoides var. capri	ATPase	Native (cholesterol)	No break		302
		Adapted (–cholesterol)	18		302

A. laidlawii (grown on 18:0)	ATPase	– Cholesterol	18	151
		+ Cholesterol	11	
Sarcoplasmic reticulum	ATPase	...	20	303
Sarcoplasmic reticulum	ATPase (isolated)	Reconstituted with dioleyl lecithin	30	59
E. coli	Proline transport	+ Elaidate	26	304
		+ Oleate	19	
		+ Linoleate	14	
E. coli	β–galactoside and β–glucoside transport	+ Elaidate	30	305
		+ β–Br–stearate	22	
		+ Oleate	13	
		+ Dehydrosterculate	11	
		+ cis–Vaccenate	10	
		+ Linoleate	7	
Erythrocytes	Acetylcholinesterase	EFA–sufficient	20	306
		EFA–deficient	28	
Mitochondria	ATPase	...	16–20	29, 282
		Butanol	No break	
		Ether	12	
		Methoxyflurane	15	

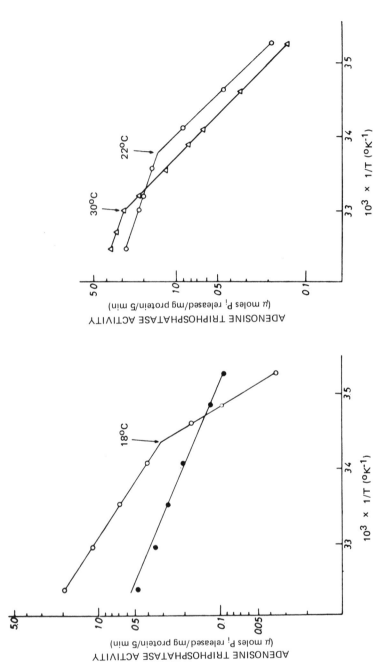

FIG. 22 Left: Arrhenius plots of ATPase activity of membranes of the native and adapted M. mycoides cells grown in a medium containing palmitic and oleic acids. ●——●, membranes of the native strain (containing high cholesterol); ○——○, membranes of the adapted strain (containing low cholesterol). Right: Arrhenius plots of ATPase activity of membranes of the adapted cells grown in a medium containing palmitic and oleic acids (○——○) or palmitic and elaidic acids (△——△). Reproduced from Rottem et al. [302], with kind permission of Elsevier Publishing Company.

Ca^{2+} ATPase from sarcoplasmic reticulum was reconstituted with dioleyl lecithin by a lipid-substitution technique; even if the phase transition of this lecithin is at -22 °C, the break of ATPase activity was found at +29 °C. Here a striking correlation was found, however, with the transient cluster formation beginning at about 30 °C in dioleyl lecithin bilayers, as detected by partitioning of TEMPO [59].

In some studies, different activities from the same membrane show breaks at different temperatures [300, 306, 310], suggesting the specific association of lipids having different fluidities. The fluidity of a membrane can be modified, however, by assay conditions (presence of extrinsic proteins, such as excess cytochrome c, or metal ions, or pH differences). We have found [unpublished] that cytochrome c lowers the discontinuity of ATPase activity in submitochondrial particles by 6 °C.

In membranes containing cholesterol, the temperature dependence shows breaks at different behavior in accordance with the effect of cholesterol on fluidity. In membranes of Mycoplasma mycoides var. capri adapted to grow with low cholesterol concentrations, the native strain (high cholesterol) has no lipid transition and no breaks in Arrhenius plots of ATPase activity [302]. On the other hand, the adapted strain (low cholesterol) shows a break in lipid fluidity at 24 °C and a sharp break at 18 °C for ATPase activity (Fig. 22). In A. laidlawii, De Kruyff et al. [151] found that adding cholesterol decreases the break temperature of ATPase and the temperature of the lower phase of the calorimetric transition.

In conclusion, the physical state of membrane lipids affects the activity of membrane-bound enzymes. Phase separation that accompanies temperature-induced transitions in complex lipid mixtures induces intrinsic protein aggregation and perhaps extrusion of proteins out of the hydrophobic core of the membrane, as shown by freeze-fracture microscopy. Changes in quaternary structure and therefore in environment of enzymes having certain peptide portions anchored into the lipid bilayer may induce localized conformational changes in the active site, affecting enzyme kinetics.

VIII. EFFECT OF LIPIDS ON PROTEIN CONFORMATION:
       STRUCTURAL STUDIES

Protein conformation in macromolecules is ideally studied by X-ray diffraction but has limited application in membrane studies. Optical rotation measurements, in particular optical rotatory dispersion (ORD) and circular dichroism (CD), however, have been used extensively for investigating the conformation of macromolecules and membranes. Indeed, no other method (except IR spectroscopy and indirect tools such as spin labels and enzyme kinetics) has given such useful indications in establishing secondary structure of the component proteins in membranes as CD spectroscopy has.

Circular dichroism measures the wavelength dependence of the differential absorption of right and left beam of circularly polarized light, thus

directly probing molecular asymmetry. Several reviews are available on
optical activity (CD and ORD) of polypeptides, proteins, and biomembranes
[311-316]. In dealing with optical spectroscopy data for biomembranes that
contain several or many proteins, one must consider that the information
yielded is the average protein conformation for all the proteins in the membrane. For this reason, only isolating and purifying individual membrane
proteins will give the final answers on membrane conformation, although
much information has been recently obtained by bulk studies in intact
membranes.

The greatest problem in the last few years has been recognizing and
correcting optical artifacts in studying particulate systems like biomembranes. The artifacts arise, as Urry and Ji first recognized [317], from
light scattering, absorption dampening, and differential light scattering.
The optical rotation patterns of biological membranes, namely low amplitude
and red-shifted extrema, when compared with proteins in solution, are primarily due to such artifacts [318-323]. Several attempts have been made to
correct for the distortions and achieve meaningful CD and ORD data. Some
approaches are based on Mie scattering functions [324]. Urry and coworkers
[312, 319, 325, 326] have proposed a pseudo-reference state approach using
poly-L-glutamic acid as a model. This approach has been adopted [327], but
corrections must be applied with great caution in order not to introduce
additional artifacts.

Greenfield and Fasman [328] have given equations to resolve the spectra
into contributions due to alpha-helix, beta-structure, and random coil; the
same equations could be used for membrane proteins, but one should be
aware that different conformations from those cited above could be present
in membranes. There are other approaches to studying the conformation of
proteins in a membrane. Infrared spectroscopy has been used to probe the
conformation of plasma membranes [329] and mitochondrial membranes
[330-332]. Also, studies with fluorescent probes, like ANS [333], have suggested conformational changes in mitochondrial membranes, for example as
the result of energization conditions; for a detailed consideration of using
fluorescent probes as indicators of energy conservation, see Ref. 79.

Once correlations are applied for the particulate nature of the membranes,
alpha-helical structure appears to predominate, and not beta-structure, as
proposed in the unit membrane hypothesis [334].

Beef-heart mitochondria sonicated in order to reduce particle size, and
corrected as discussed above [319], show CD spectra that closely resemble
those of polypeptides in alpha-helical conformation (Fig. 23), with a calculated content of alpha-helix around 50%, and very little beta-structure [cf.
also 335].

Many optical rotation studies of erythrocyte ghosts have been reported
[321, 324, 325, 336, 337]. After correction with the pseudo-reference state,
the CD spectra indicate 50% alpha-helix content. Similar values were obtained
for rat-liver plasma membranes [326], whereas sarcotubular vesicles from

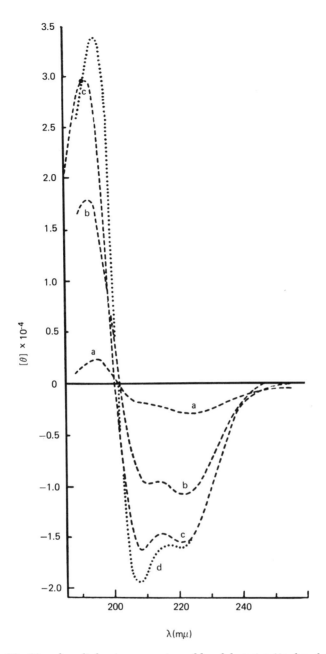

FIG. 23 Circular dichroism spectra of beef-heart mitochondria, showing the effect of sonication (b) and the corrections (d) using the pseudo-reference state (c). Reproduced from Urry et al. [325], with kind permission of Elsevier Publishing Company.

rabbit skeletal muscle are characterized by lower ellipticities, and therefore lower alpha-helix content. The lowest ellipticity was found for axonal membranes [338].

Also conformational changes during functional activity of certain membranes have been detected by CD [cf. 29].

Few optical rotation studies are available on the effect of lipids on model proteins or polypeptides, although CD spectroscopy has been widely applied to the study of serum lipoproteins.

Ulmer et al. [339] found that lipid binding has no effect on the conformation of cytochrome c, while Gulik-Krzywicki et al. [340] observed large differences in optical activity of the Soret band, which were ascribed to stacking of the heme group in the oriented bilayer systems. A very interesting model study has been reported by Letellier and Shechter [341]. Circular dichroism in the Soret region shows that adding lipids to ferricytochrome c leads to a structural change from a native to an intermediate state (displacement of the sixth ligand of the heme iron side chain of Met-80), while no structural change of ferrocytochrome c is induced by lipid binding. In the presence of lipids, the reduction of cytochrome c is accompanied by a drastic structural change from the "intermediate" ferricytochrome c to the "native" ferrocytochrome c. Complexing cytochrome c with phospholipids stabilizes the protein against denaturation [342].

The best evidence available that lipids modify the protein environment, thus inducing conformational changes, comes from studies of serum lipoproteins. Several studies [343-345] have shown that human plasma high-density lipoproteins (HDL) have a helical content of about 60%, but delipidation decreases the alpha-helix content while increasing disordered structure [345, 346]; readdition of lipids restores the native alpha-helix content to different extents depending on the nature of the lipid [345, 347, 348]. More recently, studies with the purified components have been able to show which parts of the apoproteins bind lipids and are more directly involved in the changes in conformation caused by binding [349, 350].

A similar analysis has been reported for very low density lipoproteins. Titration of apolipoprotein-Ala [351] with a sonicated dispersion of PC increases the calculated alpha-helical content from 22% to 54%, with maximal helicity at a stoichiometry of 50 PC : 1 ApoLP-Ala. An analysis of the helix-forming ability of each amino acid residue [352] leads to the conclusion that while the intrinsic helicity should be 29%, phospholipids provide the forces necessary to increase this value about twofold.

The Folch-Lees proteolipid [353], which in water has a helical content of 42%, becomes almost 100% alpha-helical in hydrophobic solvents [354] and significantly when recombined with a mixture of 1 PC : 1 cholesterol [355]. Stability of hydrophobic (intrinsic) proteins is best assured by the highest possible number of interpeptide hydrogen bonds, which occurs by forming alpha helixes in hydrophobic media such as lipids. Accordingly, it is proposed that the hydrophobic segment of the MN glycoprotein (the portion that spans the erythrocyte membrane) is alpha-helical [356].

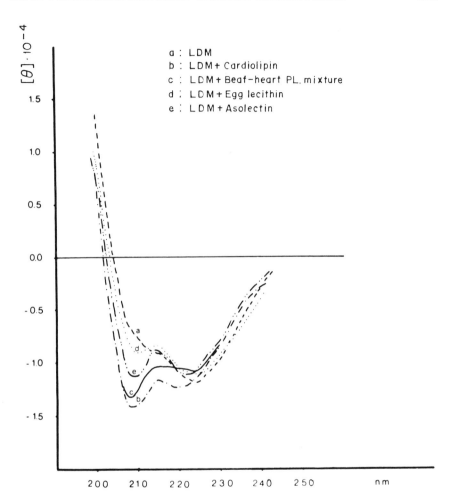

FIG. 24 Circular dichroism of mitochondrial membranes depleted and reconstituted by addition of different phospholipids; the curves are corrected for light scattering, absorption dampening, and differential light scattering. Reproduced from Masotti et al. [360], with kind permission of Academic Press.

Removal of as little as 1% of the original lipid in Ca^{2+} ATPase from the sarcoplasmic reticulum causes a reduction in helical content from 35% to 28% [357]. Extracting large quantities of lipids, however, does not alter the CD spectra significantly, while removal of DOC restores the original CD pattern. The study is complicated by using detergent, which may itself induce conformational alterations.

Several membranes have been treated with phospholipases to assess the contribution of lipids to their optical rotation spectra. Treating erythrocyte

ghosts with phospholipase C shows that the phosphate group has no effect on
protein conformation [358], and phospholipase C treatment of Ehrlich ascite
carcinoma cells [336] induces enhancement of the distortions characteristic
of membranes (lower amplitude and red-shifted extrema), indicating the
occurrence of aggregation following removal of superficial charged groups.
In contrast, ghosts treated with phospholipase A or lysolecithin show CD
spectra characterized by higher magnitude of the 208-nm and 192-nm bands
[336], in this case indicating reduction of particle size of the membrane
fragments. In submitochondrial particles (which are already small because
of sonication) changes in secondary structure after phospholipase A treatment were not observed [359]. On the other hand, Masotti et al. [360] have
found that acetone-extracted mitochondria show largely modified CD spectra
in comparison with original mitochondria; adding different phospholipids,
however, brings back the original conformation. The modification of spectra
by lipid depletion includes an exaggeration of the red shift and a disappear-
ance of the band at 208 nm. The spectra of lipid-depleted mitochondria
remain substantially different from the spectra of intact mitochondria or
lipid-reconstituted mitochondria even after corrections are applied for the
particulate nature of the samples, indicating that the changes are not the
results of aggregation but depend on conformational changes of the mitochondrial proteins. The original CD patterns of intact mitochondria (corrected
for the artifacts) were restored to different extents by different phospholipids, cardiolipin being the most effective (Fig. 24).

The differences in the results of Masotti et al. [360] and Zahler et al.
[359] can be explained by the difference in procedure used for delipidation as
well as by inability of phospholipase A to extract those phospholipids that are
more tightly associated to membrane proteins, and these are probably the
ones essential for modulating membrane protein conformation.

IX. PROTEIN-LIPID INTERACTIONS STUDIED WITH ISOLATED PROTEINS

Until recently, most studies on lipid-protein interactions were accomplished
using proteins that are not true candidates for lipid binding in vivo [30]. The
reason for such choice was mainly because true intrinsic proteins were not
available for such studies. These investigations, however, are worthy of
analysis for various reasons. First of all, they have established model systems and strategies for the study of lipid-protein associations. Second, they
have sometimes given information on the binding of extrinsic proteins to the
membranes. Moreover, they have shown that even for relatively simple systems different types of interactions may occur, with a variety of dynamic
effects (permeability, etc.) on the membranes.

A. Basic Proteins and Peptides

Protein interaction has been studied with monolayer, black lipid membranes, and bilayer vesicles [361]. The older studies have been reviewed in detail previously [30] and will be only summarized here.

Most studies were accomplished by causing basic proteins (polylysine, lysozyme, cytochrome c etc.) or proteins below their isoelectric point to interact with the lipid systems. In monolayers, interaction could be detected by variations of surface radioactivity or by actually measuring the amount of protein that had left the aqueous subphase [6, 362, 363]. These results together were compatible with an initial electrostatic attraction between positively charged proteins and anionic lipids, followed by hydrophobic interaction and penetration of the monolayers by the proteins, forming packages alternated with packages of lipid. Penetration occurs only at low initial surface pressures, while at increasing pressures the proteins are ejected into the subphase, this ejection requiring NaCl in the case of acidic phospholipids [364].

Similar conclusions were reached for the binding of basic proteins to phospholipid vesicles and although mere electrostatic interactions were first considered to be important in the binding [169, 365-367], it was later evident that hydrophobic stabilization of the complexes could occur also in bilayer systems. In the system lysozyme-cardiolipin, two principal lamellar phases were observed by Gulik-Krzywicki et al. [340]. In the so called phase III, the thickness of the lipid leaflet is the same as in lipid-water, whereas in phase IV a shrinkage of the lipid was interpreted to involve hydrophobic contacts of protein with the lipid molecules. The "hydrophobic" phase and the "electrostatic" phase could also be differentiated by using fluorescent probes like ANS and dansyl-PE. In the hydrophobic phases, the microenvironment of the probe is of lower polarity and ANS appears in closer contact with the protein [368, 369].

Kimelberg and Papahadjopoulos [363, 370] have suggested that many other proteins after an initial ionic attraction can penetrate the interior of anionic phospholipids with subsequent hydrophobic stabilization. This suggestion is supported by the very sensitive relation of the type of interaction with ion permeability. Lysozyme, cytochrome c, and albumin at acidic pH interact with phospholipid vesicles and enhance $^{22}Na^+$ permeability in accord with their penetration of PS liposomes. Similar conclusions were also reached by Dawson [241] on the reaction of phospholipases at the lipid-water interface. The demonstration of enzyme activity implies that the enzyme has approached the interface and has become stereochemically locked with the phospholipid. The reaction of phospholipases requires definite electrostatic conditions (for example, a positive zeta potential for phospholipase C). The complete interaction may, however, involve hydrogen and hydrophobic bonds of the protein side chains penetrating spaces between the lipid molecules. More recent studies with pancreatic phospholipase A_2 [242, 243] have suggested the existence of a specific "penetration site," a hydrophobic sequence distinct

from the active site; only penetration of this sequence allows optimal alignment of the active site. According to this view, the zymogen has the active
site but lacks the penetration site.

Cytolytic bacterial toxins interact with membranes [371] and in certain
cases their site of action may be phospholipids, as suggested by studies of
the interaction of cationic staphylococcal α-toxin with lipid monolayers [372].
Also, the lytic amphipathic cationic peptide melitin has been used as a model
of lipid-protein interactions. The initial ionic interaction must be followed by
hydrophobic association and penetration since the peptide affects motion of
stearic acid spin labels [373] and of a cholestane probe [374].

The interaction of α_{s1}-casein and K-casein with lysolecithin is hydrophobic as probed by PMR and spin labeling [375] with little contributions of
the polar heads of the lipids. The micellar organization of lysolecithin appears
preserved on interaction.

Studies have also been conducted on the interaction of synthetic peptides
or polypeptides with monolayers and bilayers [376-381]. Polyamino acids
may be useful in studying the role of specific amino acid side chains. Surface
pressure changes and binding of labeled polyamino acids to monomolecular
films have been studied with combination of 16 different polyamino acids and
11 different films [381]. In general, pressure changes occurred only when
basic peptides interacted with negative lipid films, but significant binding of
labeled polylysine to lipid films with no net charge could be measured in the
absence of accompanying pressure changes. It was calculated that polylysine
could bind to PC by intertwining among the phosphorylcholine groups without
distorting overall film properties. In several other cases, increase of surface
pressure involved hydrophobic binding. The studies with phospholipid bilayers
were followed by reduction in bilayer resistance accompanying hydrophobic
penetration.

Also anionic polyamino acids like polyglutamic acid have been bound to
phospholipid vesicles (PC, having no net charge) [382, 383].

The interaction of brain lipid multibilayers with different proteins and
peptides was investigated by Butler et al. [18], using proteins of known
physical properties, amino acid composition, and sequence, and evaluating
the degree of anisotropy in ESR spectra of spin labels. A first group of proteins (lysozyme, ribonuclease A, trypsin, ovomucoid, chymotrypsynogen,
insulin) interacted predominantly electrostatically with the multibilayers and
induced high degrees of organization, while others had lower ordering effects
and some (haptoglobin 1-1, lysine-phenylalanine copolymer, gelatin) had
disordering effects attributed to hydrophobic intercalation of amino acid side
chains into the lipid bilayers. With synthetic copolymers, it was found that
Phe, Ala, and Leu residues in addition to Lys led to disorder, and that they
could cross the bilayers by hydrophobic penetration, exerting their effects
beyond the first few bilayers. The effect of copolymers of Lys-Ala or Lys-
Phe depends on the absolute concentration of Ala or Phe, while copolymers
of Lys-Leu had effects depending on the ratio of the two amino acids.

Gitler and Montal [200, 201] have studied the effect on lipid-protein inter-action of protonation of protein acidic groups and of their neutralization by cations. It was shown that cytochrome c and other proteins in the presence of a mixture of phospholipids with a net negative charge could not be extracted into decane unless the proteins' carboxylic acid groups were neutralized by protonation or by adding different salts. It was theorized that the acidic phospholipids formed ion pairs with the protein cationic residues and when the proteins' carboxylic acid groups were neutralized, the overall complex became hydrophobic and could partition into the apolar solvent. The ion pairing may be very efficient for amphipathic molecules [384], since free energy of ion pair formation in water increases from G = <-1 cal/mole to G = -8.4 kcal/mole, when the interacting ions possess long hydrocarbon chains of 12 carbon atoms. Ca^{2+} binding allows hydrophobic interaction with lipids of Ca^{2+}-binding proteins [385, 386].

B. Extrinsic Membrane Proteins

1. Cytochrome c

The studies with cytochrome c already reported may be relevant to the physiological state of the mitochondrial inner membrane since cytochrome c is considered an extrinsic protein located on the outer side of the inner mem-brane. The location and binding of cytochrome c in vivo has been reviewed by Nicholls [387].

Owing to its soluble character, and its importance in electron transport, cytochrome c has been extensively studied. Ivanevitch et al. [388] have cor-related the methods of extraction of cytochrome c in vivo with those destabil-izing the complex of cytochrome c with mitochondrial phospholipids.

Further studies on monolayers [389] have confirmed that penetration by cytochrome c occurs, and a dominant factor is the expanded character of the film, which can be related to unsaturation of the lipids in bilayer membranes.

The most effective lipid that binds cytochrome c is phosphatidic acid (4 to 5 molecules needed to complex one cytochrome c), while other anionic lipids require about ten charges for binding one cytochrome molecule [390-393]. Cytochrome c binding to cardiolipin has been studied by the fluorescence quenching of 12-(9-anthroyl) stearic acid [394] and the binding has been shown to be biphasic.

Like other basic proteins, cytochrome c can be extracted into organic solvents like isooctane or ether in the presence of anionic phospholipids [365, 395, 396]. According to Gitler and Montal [200], formation of ion pairs allows partition of the cytochrome c-phospholipid complex in decane. The structure of the lipid-cytochrome c complex in organic solvents is probably an inverted micelle [395] with molecular weight about 1.3×10^6 [366].

Ivanevitch et al. [342] have studied the binding of oxidized and reduced cytochrome c to mitochondrial phospholipids. The marked decrease of

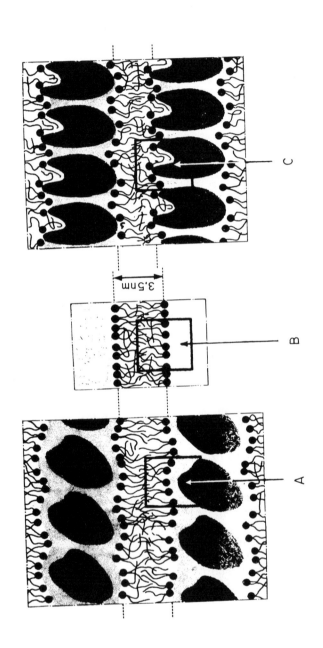

FIG. 25 Structure of the lamellar phases of cytochrome c-cardiolipin-water systems. The densely and lightly hatched areas represent the protein molecules and the water regions. (A) Lamellar phase of electrostatic type (ferricytochrome c); (B) lamellar cardiolipin-water phase; (C) lamellar phase of the hydrophobic type (ferro-cytochrome c), with decreased thickness of the lipid. Reproduced from Letellier and Shechter [341], with kind permission of the Federation of European Biochemical Societies.

exchange of the complexed cytochrome $\underline{c}$ with exogenous cytochrome $\underline{c}$ by Fe^{3+} reduction indicates that ferrocytochrome $\underline{c}$ binds more firmly to mixed phospholipids than ferricytochrome $\underline{c}$. Phospholipids are able to change the conformation of ferricytochrome $\underline{c}$ but not of the reduced protein. Similar conclusions were reached by Letellier and Shechter [341] by examining the correlation existing between fluorescence of dansyl PE and type of interaction. Electrostatic interaction was found for ferricytochrome $\underline{c}$ and hydrophobic interaction for ferrocytochrome c (Fig. 25). Accordingly, the complex is dissociated by salt only in the case of oxidized cytochrome. As discussed already, CD in the Soret region shows that phospholipid addition to ferri-cytochrome $\underline{c}$ leads to a structural change, while no structural change is seen for reduced $\underline{c}$.

2. Spectrin

Spectrin is an extrinsic protein complex located on the inner side of the erythrocyte membrane. Spectrin interacts with phospholipid vesicles and penetrates phospholipid monolayers but only at low pH [397]. However, Ca^{2+} promotes spectrin-vesicle interaction at physiological pH, causing profound changes in Na^+ permeability. The explanation suggested for the effect of Ca^{2+} is formation of a tridentate complex in which anionic sites on the protein and on the vesicles are the ligands for Ca^{2+}. Ion pairs as proposed by Gitler and Montal [200] could well explain these results.

3. Soluble Enzymes

Dodd [262] has studied the interaction of glutamate dehydrogenase and malate dehydrogenase with phospholipid membranes. Although binding of malate dehydrogenase seems to indicate, by NMR studies, that both polar and apolar interactions are involved, with glutamate dehydrogenase the main determinant of complex formation seems the charge of the lipid headgroup. Interaction is accompanied by loss of enzyme activity as discussed already. Maximal binding occurs with cardiolipin vesicles, and the interaction decreases with increasing ionic strength.

4. A_1 Myelin Basic Protein

Myelin is a simplified plasma membrane with no glycoprotein and only three significant components: the Folch-Lees proteolipid, the Wolfgram protein, and the basic A_1 protein [398]. The A_1 protein (30% of the total pro-tein) can be prepared in highly soluble homogeneous form [399] and its interest depends on its activity in inducing experimental allergic encephalo-myelitis, an autoimmune disease similar to human demyelinating diseases. The sequence of A_1 (170 amino acids) has been determined [400] and the basic residues (25% of total) were found randomly distributed over the entire poly-peptide chain, suggesting the importance of ionic interactions in the binding [398].

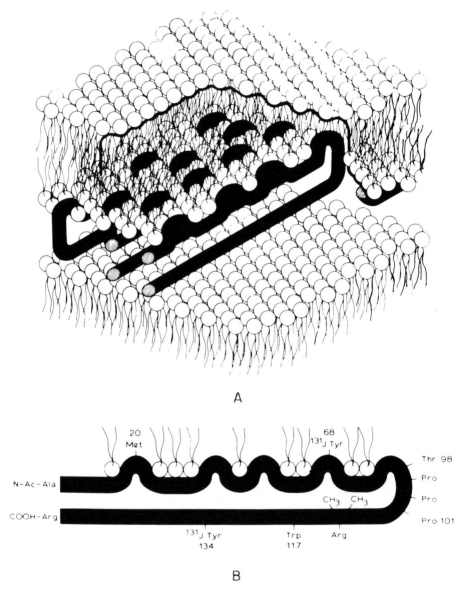

A

B

FIG. 26 Schematic representation of (A) the specific binding sites and
(B) conformation of the A_1 basic protein from myelin after complex formation
with lipids. Reproduced from London et al. [403], with kind permission of
Elsevier Publishing Company.

Knowledge of the amino acid sequence in A_1 has prompted studies directed to understanding specific binding sites with the lipids. London and Vossenberg [401] have found that specific regions of the A_1 sequence were protected from the hydrolytic action of trypsin only after the protein was recombined with specific lipids. The order of protection was cerebroside sulfate > acidic lipids from myelin > PS = total myelin lipids. The protected Lys-X, Arg-X bonds were all situated in the region 20 → 113 of the intact protein. This region contains a (proline)$_3$ bend (99 → 101) in the protein that is stabilized by interaction with lipids, and also the encephalitogenic site for monkey and for rabbit (residues 45-90). It was suggested that sulfatides are the physiological binding sites for A_1.

Demel et al. [402] and London et al. [403] have further studied the A_1 binding with lipid monolayers at the air-water interface, showing that both ionic and hydrophobic forces are involved in the interaction. Proteolytic degradation of the A_1-lipid complex at the air-water interface confirmed that specific regions of the protein are protected after interaction with the lipids. The A_1-sulfatide complex was collected from the interface after tryptic hydrolysis, and peptide maps showed that the N-terminal portion (residues 20 → 113) is preserved in the lipid phase. All these studies suggest a model for the folded molecule in which only the N-terminal portion interacts with lipids. The N-terminus contains more nonpolar amino acids than the C-terminus (117 → 170), suggesting that nonpolar hydrophobic associations are also important. Figure 26 gives a schematic representation of the specific binding of A_1 with the lipid bilayer. The specific association of A_1 with negative lipids, together with the fact that Folch-Lees apoprotein reacts preferentially with cholesterol, suggests that the myelin membrane is asymmetric, and asymmetry is specifically directed by the protein. A working hypothesis was advanced that A_1 is the organizer molecule that initiates the spiral winding of myelin around the axon. The basic protein extruded from the myelin membrane will cause an asymmetric charge distribution to give a more polar external side of the membrane, while the Folch-Lees apoprotein by its different lipid specificity will cause asymmetric distribution of cholesterol, PE, and sphingomyelin, resulting in a more hydrophobic cytoplasmic side. The asymmetry will cause the myelin mechanically to wrap around the axon.

As for the origin of the basic protein during myelin formation, it is of interest that the protein moiety of the major glycoprotein from sciatic nerve contains a sequence similar to that of the basic proteins of peripheral nerve system myelin [404-406].

5. Effect of Extrinsic Proteins on Lipid Fluidity

Few studies are available on the effect that peripheral proteins have on the fluidity of lipid bilayers. Cytochrome c and other basic proteins (lysozyme, polylysine) lower the phase transition temperature of phospholipids by 10 °C

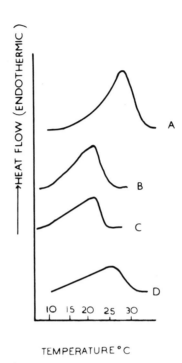

FIG. 27 Differential scanning calorimetry heating curves of (A) PS :
water (50:50) ($T_t = 28$ °C); (B) PS–cytochrome c : water (50 : 50) ($T_t = 21$ °C);
(C) PS–lysozyme : water (50 : 50) ($T_t = 21.5$ °C); (D) PS–polylysine : water
(50 : 50) ($T_t = 25$ °C). Reproduced from Chapman et al. [37], with kind permission of the American Society of Biological Chemists.

[37, 407] (Fig. 27). The shifted transition is probably related to the reorgan-
ization of the polar groups by ionic interaction with the charged groups of the
proteins in fixed positions, leading to less efficient packing of the lipid chains.
The effect is opposite to that given by cations, possibly as a result of their
charges being mobile and not restricted as in proteins. Basic proteins also
appear to restrict the mobility of fatty acyl chains locally, as detected by
spin-labeling. A spin-label study using 5-, 12-, and 16-doxyl stearic acid
has shown that the basic proteins immobilize only the probe having the nitroxide nearest to the polar heads, while no effect is apparent for the other labels
[70]. It is likely that basic proteins immobilize the neighboring segments of
the lipid chains but at the same time decrease the overall packing of the fatty
chains in the bilayer, leading to decreased transition temperature.

In contrast, Verkleij et al. [38] found that the A_1 basic protein from
myelin increases the transition temperature as studied by DSC. Also Bertoli
et al. [408] have found that the phase transition temperatures (measured by

DSC) in promitochondrial membranes from S. cerevisiae are higher than those in lipid extracts, and have related these differences to "polar" interactions of lipids with proteins. Polar interactions would lead in this case to more efficient packing of the lipids. Such differences do not usually occur in membranes [37] or are quantitatively small [42], arguing against the importance of polar interactions in most membrane systems.

In a recent study, Papahadjopoulos et al. [409] have studied a variety of proteins for their ability to interact and alter the thermotropic properties of phospholipid membranes as detected by DSC. The interactions were grouped in three categories. Proteins of group 1 (ribonuclease and polylysine) show strong electrostatic binding and increase the enthalpy of transition with either an increase or no change in the transition temperature. Group 2 proteins (cytochrome c and A_1 myelin basic protein) also show electrostatic binding but decrease both ΔH and temperature of transition. Group 3 proteins (myelin proteolipid and gramicidin A) induce a decrease of ΔH but have no effect on transition temperatures. It was concluded that Group 2 proteins partially penetrate the bilayer with deformation of the bilayer itself, while Group 3 proteins effect complete penetration, with hydrophobic binding to a limited number of lipid molecules, leaving the rest of the bilayer unperturbed.

C. Intrinsic Membrane Proteins

1. Protein Penetration and the Fraction of Lipid That Is in Contact with Intrinsic Proteins

A point to clarify for intrinsic proteins is the extent of hydrophobic contact between lipids and proteins in an intact membrane. The problem in the early times was whether there is hydrophobic contact of the nonpolar fatty chains with parts of protein molecules. It is now quite well established that protein penetration of the lipids occurs in membrane structure and the problem is shifted to the extent of contact between protein and fatty acid. Let us consider first what evidence we have that protein penetration is one of the main features of membrane structure.

The demonstration that hydrophobic interactions between lipids and proteins are important in membrane structure [30] is not a sufficient reason per se to prove that integral proteins become deeply immersed in the lipid bilayer [30, 182] because other relations may be compatible with such kind of interaction. On the other hand, the following findings are in favor of extensive penetration of several membranes by proteins [410].

1. The polar heads of membrane lipids are equally available to phospholipase attack or to interaction with basic proteins as the same groups in pure bilayer lipids [84, 390]. Träuble and Overath [81] have compared the amount of lipids that take part in the thermotropic transition in membranes and protein-free lipids, as measured by ANS fluorescence. Since ANS binds the bilayer surface at least in part ionically, the fraction of lipids that takes part

in the transition corresponds to that available to interaction with ANS, that is, those not bound to extrinsic proteins (42.5% of total lipids).

2. Specific nonpenetrating protein reagents demonstrate that certain proteins or protein complexes span the whole membrane thickness, since they are available from both sides of the same membranes [411].

3. Immobilization of lipid fatty acid chains by proteins is operative even at the level of the deepest methylene groups in the case of intrinsic membrane proteins, while extrinsic proteins affect mainly the most superficial methylenes [70].

4. Freeze-fracture electron microscopy has shown particles embedded in the lipid bilayer, and these particles are unambiguously demonstrated as protein in nature [412].

5. Several techniques have shown lateral mobility and rotation of intrinsic membrane proteins in fluid bilayers [cf. 29].

In addition, functional criteria related to the mechanisms of energy conservation in energy-transducing membranes and to the molecular basis of transport have suggested a protein continuity across a given membrane long before that continuity could be established on a structural basis.

Once it is firmly established that lipid alkyl chains are in contact with proteins, it is important to determine the extent of contact and the fraction of lipid directly bound to proteins.

Vanderkooi [195] has calculated the extent of contact in the case of cytochrome oxidase, from the experimental findings of electron microscopy and from the fraction of lipids that is immobilized by the protein components [413]. Assuming for cytochrome oxidase protein a minimum molecular weight about 200,000 and assuming an average phospholipid content 26.5% by weight (in the isolated oxidase without lipid addition), and a molecular weight per lipid phosphorus of 775, a ratio of 93 molecules of phospholipid per protein complex is obtained [195]. In the lattice structure appearing when this preparation is viewed by electron microscopy, the half-unit cell area is 5,000 $\mathring{A}^2$ from the optical transform [414]; of this area approximately 3,000 $\mathring{A}^2$ is occupied by the white spot presumed to be protein, with 2,000 $\mathring{A}^2$ remaining for the lipid, corresponding to 43 $\mathring{A}^2$ per lipid molecule in a bilayer structure.

The lipid content of cytochrome oxidase can, however, be artificially varied from a very low content to a maximum of 0.7 mg lipid per mg protein [415]. The crystalline structure to which the above calculations were referred was found in the range of 0.33–0.43 mg lipid per mg protein [195]. The morphology is amorphous at lower lipid, while proteins are randomly distributed for higher lipid content. The fact that above 0.7 mg per mg no further dilution of proteins is possible indicates that the proteins must still have attractive forces limiting infinite mixing with lipids.

The spin-label studies of cytochrome oxidase at increasing lipid content [413] indicate progressive increase of motional freedom from a highly immobilized state in the lipid-poor protein. Computer analysis of digitalized spectra has shown that the experimental spectra are due to the contribution of a class of immobilized bound lipids and a class of free bilayer lipids (fluid) appearing above 0.2 mg lipid per mg protein. The results indicated that on lipidation the amount of bound lipids remains essentially constant but the amount of free component increases. A rough calculation shows that 0.2 mg lipid per mg protein corresponds to 52 molecules of lipid per molecule of protein, based on the previous assumptions for molecular weights. Assuming a surface area of 40 Å^2 per bound lipid molecule, Jost et al. [413, 416] calculated that only one layer around the protein is strongly immobilized "boundary" lipid.

From the above considerations, it can be roughly evaluated that at maximum lipidation, one third of the membrane is occupied by protein and two thirds by lipids. Of the lipids, only 25%–30% must be directly bound to the protein, and the rest is free bilayer (Fig. 28).

These figures for cytochrome oxidase are the best values available for a membrane system, but agree quite well with investigations in which the extent of contact was established by other means.

Differential scanning calorimetry has shown that approximately 25% of phospholipids in mitochondrial and A. laidlawii membranes [42, 417] do not undergo the calorimetric transition. If these lipids correspond to the strongly immobilized layer, where the lipids are forced not to assume a crystalline arrangement even at low temperatures by the constraints imposed by proteins [29], then the agreement seems very good.

Träuble and Overath [81] have compared the fluorescence of N-phenyl-1-naphthylamine (NPN) in E. coli membranes and isolated lipids (Fig. 29); the fluorescence change ΔI at the phase transition approaches a limiting value ΔI_{lim} with increasing dye concentration. A comparison of limiting values ΔI_{lim} obtained for membranes and protein-free lipids allows estimating the lipid fraction in the membrane that takes part in the phase transition (80%). Calculation from these values gives an average of about 600 lipid molecules surrounding each integral protein. Of these lipid molecules, 130 appear to be closely coupled to the protein molecule, forming a halo in which the chain-chain interaction between the lipids is disturbed.

These values agree with similar results obtained by spin–labeling [418, 419] and by X-ray crystallography [420–423]. The amount of protein interrupting a lipid bilayer may be estimated from the distance between lipid headgroups, provided that the volume of lipid unit area of the membrane is known. Differences of 20%–30% between calculated and measured values give the area of membrane occupied by protein.

Overath et al. [424] have directly compared X-ray and NPN fluorescence studies to calculate the amount of lipids taking part in the transition in outer and inner membranes of E. coli, and found 60%–80% in the inner membrane, but only 25%–40% in the outer membrane (in accordance with its higher protein content), with good agreement between the two methods.

Freeze–fracture electron microscopy allows direct visualization of the intrinsic proteins so that the actual area of the particles and particle–free surfaces can be measured. If it is assumed that the average diameter of

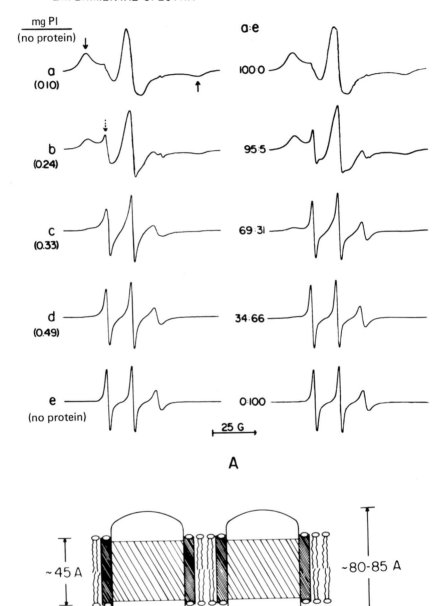

EXPERIMENTAL SPECTRA   SUMMED SPECTRA

$\dfrac{\text{mg PI}}{\text{(no protein)}}$ a:e

a
(0·10)   100·0

b
(0.24)   95·5

c
(0.33)   69:31

d
(0.49)   34·66

e
(no protein)   0·100

25 G

A

~45 A   ~80-85 A

B

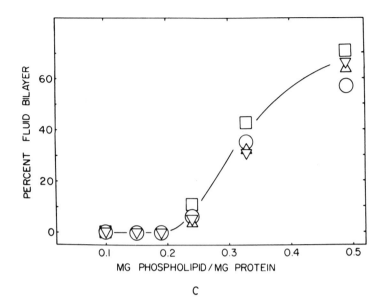

C

FIG. 28 (Left and above) Boundary lipids in cytochrome oxidase [416].
A. ESR spectra of 16-doxylstearic acid in cytochrome oxidase with varying
phospholipid content. The numbers at the left represent the phospholipid :
protein ratios. In the right column are synthesized spectra obtained by sum-
ming various amounts of spectrum a (lipid:protein ratio of 0.10) and spectrum
e (lipids extracted from membranous cytochrome oxidase) in the proportions
indicated. B. Diagrammatic cross-sectional view of membranous cytochrome
oxidase. The densely crosshatched regions represent immobilized boundary
lipid. C. Summary of calculations of percentage of fluid bilayer in cytochrome
oxidase as a function of phospholipid content. Each set represents a different
kind of calculation. Reproduced from Jost et al. [416], with kind permission
of Alan Liss Publishing Company.

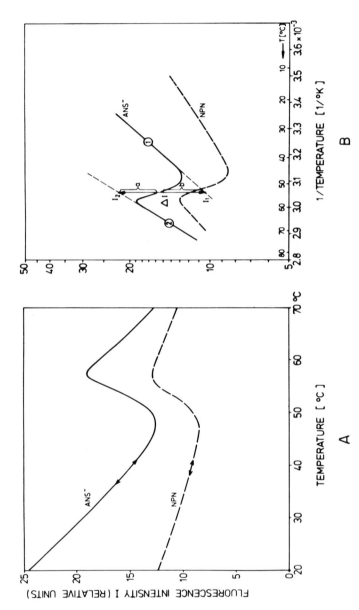

FIG. 29 Response of the fluorescence intensities of ANS⁻ and NPN to the thermal phase transition of distearoyl lecithin dispersions. A. I vs. T. B. log I vs 1/T; straight lines with different slopes are obtained for the two states (1) below and (2) above the phase transition. ΔI is defined as the difference $(I_2 - I_1)$ between the extrapolated lines at a temperature T_t, where the measured curve bisects the difference $(I_2 - I_1)$. Reproduced from Träuble and Overath [81], with kind permission of Elsevier Publishing Company.

intramembrane particles is 100 Å and there are an average of 1,000-3,000 particles per μm^2, then they make up 0.1-0.3 μm^2 that is 10%-30% of the fracture face. Even after correcting for the shadow process the valves would only be 20%-30% lower. This corrected particle area, however, does not necessarily correspond to the protein area and the uncertainty suggests caution in the interpretation of areas of proteins and lipids as calculated from electron micrographs. Freeze fracture, however, by showing that in most membranes the particle density is different in the two fracture faces, indicates that other methods may only give average values of contact for the two monolayers that the lipid bilayer comprises.

2. Lateral Mobility of Proteins within the Lipid Milieu

There is now considerable interest in the degree and nature of protein mobility in membranes. This is not surprising since problems such as energy conservation mechanisms (oxidative and photosynthetic phosphorylation) assume a different perspective if the systems are thought of as associated with fixed arrays of protein complexes or with components that are statistically free to move in the membrane. Similarly, an understanding of biological transport across membranes awaits clarification of the carrier mechanism— whether a fixed channel structure exists or a complex can freely rotate across the membrane, or both. Different types of mobility are indicated in Figure 30. It is not in the scope of this review to discuss in detail protein mobility in membranes, and the subject will be only summarized here.

Microscopic techniques and in particular freeze-etching electron microscopy have given the first indications that proteins can diffuse transversely in membranes. A characteristic feature of most membranes is the existence of particles in the fracture faces; the identification of the particles with proteins has been obtained by reconstituting lipoprotein membranes by adding proteins (for example the main erythrocyte glycoprotein) to bilayers [412]. Aggregation of intramembranous particles occurs in conjunction with phase separation of membrane lipids [425-428]. Cooling results in the squeezing out of penetrating proteins (i.e. intramembranous particles), thus resulting in the full separation of lipids and proteins. The presence of cholesterol in a membrane prevents particle aggregation, in accordance with its abolition of lipid phase separation [429]. Temperature and other agents may induce agglutination of intramembrane particles. In erythrocyte ghosts, the particles are reversibly aggregated by pH changes (optimally pH 5.5) [430], and this aggregation is accompanied by reversible aggregation of positively charged colloidal iron bound to the membrane surface [431], suggesting that the binding sites are present in intrinsic molecules capable of translational diffusion. A possible explanation may be linked to the physical properties of spectrin, an extrinsic protein bound to the inner membrane surface, which has a isoelectric point of 5.5. Spectrin molecules may interact with a segment of the MN glycoprotein [432] (a transmembrane control of cell surface

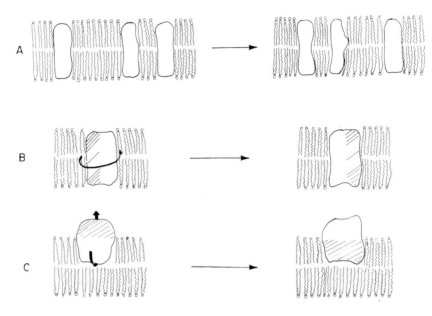

FIG. 30 Protein mobility in membranes: A. Lateral diffusion. B. Rotation in the plane of the membrane. C. Rotation perpendicular to the plane of the membrane.

topography). Spectrin may have the function of stabilizing the distribution of membrane proteins in vivo [433], and this can be a general function exerted by extrinsic proteins on intrinsic membrane proteins.

Edidin [434] has used antibodies as probes of the physical state of the cell surface and by different kinds of experiments on cultured cells has calculated diffusion coefficients for membrane proteins ranging from 10^{-9} cm^2/sec to 5×10^{-11} cm^2/sec.

There have also been physicochemical approaches to the demonstration of protein diffusion. Junge [435] has measured the depolarization of absorption of cytochrome oxidase at 445 nm by following the flash photolysis of the CO complex using linearly polarized laser light. Since no polarization could be detected, the results were interpreted to mean rapid rotation of the molecule in the membrane (see later). Since glutaraldehyde fixation induced polarization, this was taken as demonstration that proteins are free to approach each other for a sufficient fraction of time to become cross-linked by glutaraldehyde, thereby implying freedom of diffusion. The lateral diffusion of rhodopsin in frog retina has also been observed using a microspectrophotometric technique, and diffusion coefficients of the order of 4×10^{-9} to 5.5×10^{-9} cm^2/sec have been measured [436]. If the rhodopsin on one side of the membrane is suddenly bleached, the rhodopsin on the other side can be seen to diffuse rapidly until a uniform distribution is achieved [437, 438]. Lateral diffusion in human erythrocyte ghosts labeled with a fluorescent marker has been calculated at 10^{-12} cm^2/sec, a value several orders of magnitude lower than in model systems [439].

As pointed out earlier, the lack of any polarization of the 445-nm absorption of the CO-cytochrome oxidase complex in mitochondria was taken as evidence that rapid rotation occurs [435]. In retina, Cone [440] observed a transient dichroism in rhodopsin absorption with a rotational relaxation time of about 20 μsec, showing that it is free to rotate in the plane of the membrane. Razi-Naqvi et al. [441] have used a special flash photolysis apparatus to observe the polarized transient absorption spectra of photo-products of both natural chromophores and suitable probes. In contrast to protein rotation in the plane of the membrane, rotation perpendicular to the plane of the membrane (flipflop) appears difficult on thermodynamic grounds. This is due to the amphipathic nature of intrinsic proteins. Measurements using protein spin label in M. lysodeikticus membranes indicate a relaxation time of about 15 min at 24 °C [442].

3. Effect of Intrinsic Proteins on Lipid Fluidity

Chapman et al. [37] have investigated the effect of the peptide gramicidin A, which becomes inserted in the hydrophobic core of lipids and forms a channel through the bilayer [443] on the transition temperature for lipids. Gramicidin A was shown to behave like cholesterol, inducing a dramatic decrease in heat content of the endothermic peak (Fig. 31). Similar results were obtained with alamethicin [444], a peptide that also has ionic channel properties [445]. The enthalpy of transition is progressively reduced in both cases by increasing the peptide-to-lipid ratio, while the temperature of the transition is slightly lowered by both peptides. The channel-forming peptides are obviously mainly stabilized by hydrophobic interactions with the lipid chains. Hydrophobic interaction of peptides with phospholipids, as in the case of cholesterol with phospholipids, should produce complexes with loss of cooperativity in transition. Such complexes are in equilibrium with free bilayer lipids at low peptide concentrations.

As pointed out previously, in natural membranes, up to one-third of the section area is occupied by intrinsic proteins. Further, one layer of phospho-lipids, one molecule thick and amounting to 25%-30% of total phosphorus, is directly in contact with the proteins, while the remaining lipids are in free bilayer form and not in direct contact with proteins. Steim [42, 417] has found that approximately 25% of A. laidlawii phospholipids do not undergo the calorimetric transition; this evidence can be obtained calculating the difference in the enthalpy change at transition between membranes and isolated lipids (normalizing to the same lipid content).

The very broad transitions found in natural membranes suggest that as in the case of isolated lipids, phospholipids are present in a wide temperature

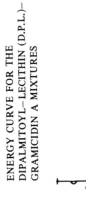

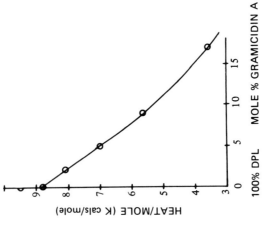

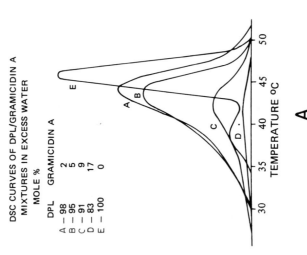

FIG. 31. A. Differential–scanning–calorimetry heating curves of dipalmitoyl PC–gramicidin A–water mixtures (50 lipid : 50 water). B. The heats of transition for dipalmitoyl PC–gramicidin A–water mixtures. Reproduced from Chapman et al. [37], with kind permission of the American Society of Biological Chemists.

range in both gel and liquid-crystalline regions, and that phase separation is a physiological feature of several membranes. Studies with A. laidlawii [417, 446] suggest that such phase separation is present even at the growth temperature of the organism. (The effect of phase separation on the protein distribution will be discussed in the next section.)

Comparison of rotational mobility of spin labels in membranes and extracted phospholipids has revealed that membrane proteins exert a strong immobilizing effect on the lipids at all depths in the bilayer [283, 447-452], in contrast with the localized effect of those proteins that bind the bilayer surface [29]. This is a further indication that intrinsic proteins are in contact with the bilayer core.

For sarcoplasmic reticulum membranes, Eletr and Inesi [453] reported two transitions probed with hydrophobic spin labels; a transition at 22 °C reflects lipid melting independently of membrane proteins, while a second transition at 40 °C disappeared after protein denaturation and was interpreted as the effect of protein conformational changes on the dynamic state of the lipids.

The increase in viscosity of lipids when they interact hydrophobically with proteins is very well documented in studies on isolated cytochrome oxidase by Jost et al. [413, 416], previously quoted. A stearic acid spin label becomes progressively more mobile as the lipid content of the complex is increased. Computer calculation shows that the mobility at any lipid content is the average of mobility of the label in the lipid-poor oxidase and in free bilayer, suggesting the existence of a strongly immobilized layer of boundary phospholipids interacting with the proteins of the complex, while the others have the same fluidity as in protein-free bilayer (Fig. 28). A steroid label confirms the above results [416], suggesting that the stearic acid label is a true indicator of the average mobility of all phospholipids. That is to say, lipids immobilized by proteins do not extrude stearic acid labels as crystalline lipids do. Immobilization by proteins is not equivalent to crystallization but is rather an increase in viscosity of a disordered lipid region. This interpretation, in accord with the previously described DSC data, is strengthened by X-ray diffraction studies. Shechter et al. [44] found that in E. coli membranes at low temperatures, the amount of ordered paraffin chains is smaller than in the corresponding lipid extract. Thus the interaction with proteins prevents ordering of lipids that have the potential of "crystallizing" in the absence of proteins. It is highly likely, then, that the strongly immobilized layer of lipids surrounding the intrinsic proteins and detected by spin-labeling does not undergo the cooperative melting of free bilayer lipids, and behaves as a disordered, yet highly viscous region in a very large temperature range. A natural membrane (not containing cholesterol) in which intrinsic proteins occupy up to 30% of the bilayer sectional area, will have the same behavior as a phospholipid bilayer containing low cholesterol and showing two phases: cholesterol-phospholipid complexes and free phospholipid bilayer. Immobilization may be more complete in membranes containing higher amounts of proteins. Esser and Lanyi [451] have found that in

H. cutirubrum membranes that have a high protein content (lipid : protein
ratio <0.2), the thermal transitions for 5- and 12-doxylstearic acid spin
labels are completely absent (as evidenced by the temperature dependence
of the order parameter S or of the rotational correlation time). On the other
hand, a thermal transition occurs in the isolated lipids. In the case of
16-doxylstearic acid, the environment may be more similar in lipids and
membranes and a thermal transition occurs in both systems. Besides
increase in the order parameter, in membranes the polarity is also higher
than in lipids, as detected by the coupling constant a'.

A complication in detecting transitions associated with intrinsic proteins
is pointed out by Bertoli et al. [408]. Cooling of membranes induces phase
separation [58] and proteins are excluded from the gel phase into the remaining fluid regions as revealed by freeze-fracture electron microscopy. Under
such conditions, the increase of protein-protein contacts will make more
lipid molecules available for lipid-lipid binding. The DSC curves of the
membrane will therefore reveal the behavior of the lipids from which the
protein has been excluded. Whether this dynamic state will much affect the
DSC data remains to be demonstrated.

4. Rhodopsin

Rhodopsin is the main component of the outer segment membranes of
retinal rods, making up 80%-90% of the total protein [454]. Rhodopsin is
associated in vivo with phospholipids, which are strikingly rich in polyunsaturated fatty acids, and especially 22 : 6 fatty acids [455, 457]. The retinal
polyunsaturated fatty acids are very resistant to dietary changes [457, 458].
The high unsaturation may be significant in protecting visual pigments from
oxidation [454]. The result of such unsaturation on the physical state of the
membrane is not, however, well known. The fluidity of the lipids and the
mobility of rhodopsin in situ have been examined [436, 438] and the architecture of the disc membrane has been studied by X-ray crystallography
[459, 461].

The lipoprotein nature of rhodopsin is now very clear. The difficulty of
extracting phospholipids from rhodopsin while leaving its function intact has
induced Poincelot et al. [462] to postulate a coenzymatic role of lipids. It
was claimed that in rhodopsin, retinaldehyde is linked to PE and this is the
physiological chromophore. However, this possibility was ruled out by mild
but extensive extraction of the phospholipids [463, 464]. The lipid-depleted
rhodopsin had spectral properties similar to those of native pigment.

How the lipids affect the properties of rhodopsin seems linked to conformational stabilization. The thermal stability of rhodopsin is decreased by lipid
depletion [465, 466], and removal of detergent by dialysis from lipid-depleted
rhodopsin results in denaturation unless dialysis is carried out in presence
of phospholipids [467]. Detergents may partly stabilize rhodopsin, but phospholipids are the natural surface-active agents that provide an ideal natural environment for the photopigment. Lipid depletion of disc membranes depresses

the regenerability of rhodopsin after photolysis to opsin, and phospholipid readdition restores the regenerability [468], probably by restoring the original stable conformation.

A functional role of phospholipid in signal transduction would demand phospholipid-rhodopsin interactions coupled to some step in bleaching of the pigment. The pressure dependence of the equilibrium between metarhodopsin I and II [469] and direct chemical observation of the intermediates [470] have shown that the lipid at metarhodopsin II is more compressible than the lipid at metarhodopsin I and this is the step in which phospholipids may be involved, perhaps in connection with conformational changes.

The successful incorporation and high regenerability of rhodopsin in phospholipid bilayers depend on the nature of the fatty acid hydrocarbon chains and not on the polar groups [471, 472], suggesting that the interaction is mainly hydrophobic and that rhodopsin penetrates the bilayer.

It was found that rhodopsin binding induces a dramatic decrease of rotational freedom of the chains (by spin-labeling) and that the protein is incorporated as discrete intramembranous particles in the plane of the membrane, as shown by freeze-etching electron microscopy. Reversible separations of pure solid lipid from rhodopsin-rich fluid phases have been observed that depend on temperature [471]. The distribution and phase behavior of the protein is altered by bleaching.

Montal and Korenbrot [473] prepared asymmetric bilayers using a technique of applying two different monolayers [13], one of glycerol dioleate and cholesterol and the other of rhodopsin proteolipid, and found that the asymmetric bilayers were more stable than symmetrical membranes of rhodopsin proteolipid. Rhodopsin incorporation reduced the membrane capacitance of the phospholipids.

The orientation of rhodopsin, already evident in studies of the molecule in situ [474] has been proved also by shearing between two quartz slides digitonin micelles of the pigment [475]. The chromophores orient parallel to the direction of shear, with the long axis parallel to the membrane at all intermediate stages of bleaching. When the retinaldehyde is hydrolyzed from opsin in the presence of hydroxylamine, the resulting oxime rotates so as to lie across the direction of shear.

5. ATPases

a. Mitochondrial ATPase. The mitochondrial Mg^{2+} ATPase, involved in oxidative phosphorylation, has been reviewed in its bioenergetic and structural aspects by Pedersen [268].

I have already described the main aspects of the allotopic properties of mitochondrial ATPase and its lipid requirement for activity and for sensitivity to energy-transfer inhibitors.

Mitochondrial ATPase has been incorporated into lipid bilayers for reconstitution of phosphorylating activities. Studies on reconstitution of oxidative phosphorylation from electron transfer complexes and ATPase lipids have already been cited. Mitochondrial electron transfer complexes were incorporated into phospholipids together with mitochondrial "hydrophobic protein" and "coupling factors" [212, 215]. It is likely that crude "hydrophobic protein" represents the intrinsic membrane factor of the mitochondria ATPase, and reconstitution of a functional ATPase complex occurs on addition of coupling factors (F_1, OSCP). According to the Mitchell hypothesis, the ATPase complex is incorporated asymmetrically across the mitochondrial inner membrane and represents a proton channel, capable of discharging the electrochemical gradient established through electron transfer across the membrane.

b. ATPase from Streptococcus faecalis. The Mg^{2+}-ATPase from S. faecalis appears to be involved in active transport of monovalent cations and other solutes across the plasma membranes [476]. The complex appears to be an intrinsic membrane protein having 12 polypeptide chains of two kinds and a molecular weight of 385,000. It was postulated [477] that it is a planar hexagonal array of six globules, each containing one α and one β subunit; the diameter of each globule is ~40 Å, and the longest dimension across the hexagon is 120 Å. A single enzyme molecule lying in the plane of the bilayer (62 Å thick) could almost span the membrane and provide a conducting pathway through the protein.

Abrams and Baron [478] studied the binding of ATPase to depleted S. faecalis ghosts and found an Mg^{2+} requirement for the association. A protein nectin, was required for sensitivity to inhibitors, but the interaction with liposomes was not impaired by increased ionic strength [479]. The ratio of PC to ATPase was 11 : 1 with a constant of association of 7.4×10^7 M^{-1}. Stearylamine increased binding at low ionic strength, while PE or cardiolipin had little effect and cholesterol lowered the binding. Lipids must be in a fluid state, and ATPase binding to dimyristoyl PC occurs above the transition temperature only. The intereaction of the ATPase appears hydrophobic, since the enthalpy change was small while the corresponding entropy contribution was 30 e.u./mole, thus providing the driving force for complex formation. The positive effect of stearylamine indicates some ionic influence on binding, while the inhibition by cholesterol appears mainly related to decreased motion of the lipids. Penetration by the protein of the bilayer is highly probable, as also indicated by the formation of larger vesicles and by broadening of high-resolution PMR signals of the choline protons [480]. The binding to black lipid membranes of diphytanoyl PC in decane was accompanied by a 10^2-fold to 10^4-fold increase of conductance (Fig. 31). At extremely low ATPase (10^{-10} M), discrete conductance fluctuations were seen [481], made up of integral multiples of a unit "channel" approximately 10^{10} Ω^{-1} in magnitude. The increased osmotic permeability and absence of ionic selectivity in the bilayer suggest that the channels are relatively wide water-filled pores. The incidence and duration of channels increased by raising the voltage, suggesting that after interaction a field-dependent transition occurs between a nonconducting and a conducting conformation [482].

6. Cytochrome b_5 and NADH-Cytochrome b_5 Reductase

Cytochrome b_5 is an electron carrier apparently involved in the micro-somal hydroxylation system. The molecule was initially obtained in soluble form by lipase or trypsin cleavage with a molecular weight of about 11,000 [483], but higher-MW forms have been obtained using detergents [484, 485]. It has been confirmed that the previously isolated soluble molecule was a proteolytic fragment of an amphipathic protein that has a hydrophobic tail anchoring the protein tightly to the membrane [484]. This extremely hydro-phobic segment of 40 amino acids is at the C terminus and is required for binding cytochrome b_5 to the liver microsome [475]. A second enzyme of the hydroxylation system, cytochrome b_5 reductase, is also amphipathic [487]. Both are randomly distributed in the microsomal membrane [489] and free to diffuse in the bilayer; a tenfold excess of the cytochrome can be bound with properties identical to endogenous b_5. There must be very high freedom of the hydrophilic parts and large flexibility at the junction so that the active site can function several times before diffusion in the lipid brings the cyto-chrome away.

Dehlinger et al. [490] have studied the interaction of spin-labeled lipids with cytochrome b_5 and found that intact b_5 immobilizes the labels, while the heme-bearing segment released by trypsin does not affect mobility. These studies confirm the existence of boundary lipids with a single membrane protein, as previously found with the multisubunit cytochrome oxidase complex [416].

Rogers and Strittmatter [491] have studied the interaction between lipid bilayers and both cytochrome b_5 and the b_5 reductase, and found that the hydrophobic portions are essential for controlling the rate of reduction of cytochrome b_5 by NADH in liver microsomes. With soluble catalytic proteins, NADH reduction of the flavin proceeds with a rate constant $k = 68$ s^{-1} and flavin reoxidation by b_5 occurs by two successive one-electron transfers with $k > 1000$ s^{-1} and 190 s^{-1} respectively. In microsomes, b_5 reduction is a much slower reaction because electron transfer subsequent to flavin reduction involves protein-protein interaction and is rate-limiting. Removal of phospho-lipids markedly decreases the rate of b_5 reduction, and reconstitution with liposomes completely restores the structural and functional characteristics of the reductase system. After removal of lipid, the enzymes are anchored to the membrane but are no longer free to diffuse and undergo collisions.

7. Myelin Proteolipid

Folch and Lees [492] described for brain a protein material soluble in chloroform-methanol mixtures and designated proteolipid. It was later found that this material in the brain is mainly associated with the myelin membrane, of which it constitutes 55% of total protein, but proteolipids have since been found in many biological membranes [353]. Purified proteolipid preparations contain about 15% lipids, mainly PS, sulfatides, and polyphosphoinositides, apparently bound by ionic linkages, which can be removed by dialysis in acidified chloroform-methanol. The proteolipid apoprotein obtained contains 2%-4% covalently bound fatty acids [353]. Careful delipidation does not alter the solubility properties in organic solvents, and ORD and CD studies using this solvent indicate a high alpha-helix content [354]. The apoprotein can be solubilized in water with a large decrease in alpha-helix content and exposure of hydrophilic groups to the medium. Dissolving the apoprotein back in chloroform-methanol regenerates the high alpha-helix content.

The protein migrates as one peak by gel electrophoresis [353], but it ma exist as a hexamer with molecular weight of about 30,000 when in association with phospholipids, while other aggregation states are possible in water with production of multiple bands [493].

The incorporation of the lipid-soluble form of the apoprotein into multi-bilayers [494] induces disorder irrespective of the net charge of the lipid molecules, whereas the aqueous form of the protein has a chaotropic effect on lipid organization only if the lipids have a net negative charge, suggesting that ionic attraction is necessary before hydrophobic stabilization (cf. Fig. 13 Examination of the ESR spectra shows that the protein alters the geometry of lipids without affecting their mobility, contrary to the results with cytochrom oxidase of Jost et al. [416].

It must be concluded that in vivo the apoprotein is necessarily combined with lipids, which constitutes a hydrophobic medium and allows a high alpha-helical content. Ion pairs with acidic groups on the surface and hydrophobic interactions in the bilayer core would greatly stabilize the proteolipid structu

London et al. [355] studied the interaction of the Folch-Lees protein with lipid monolayers and found that large changes in surface pressure were given by interaction with a variety of myelin lipids, such as cerebroside sulfate, PS, PI, PE, and cholesterol; they found that sphingomyelin, cerebroside, and PC have less affinity. Thus the proteolipid exhibits a different lipid speci ficity compared with the A_1 basic protein. The interaction with cholesterol is quite remarkable: subsequent injection of A_1 and proteolipid underneath a cholesterol monolayer shows a preferential binding of the proteolipid and rejection of A_1 from the interface. In contrast, the affinity for cerebroside sulfate is higher for A_1 basic protein. The results confirm the previously suggested penetration by the protein as well as charge interaction, with highe stability in the lipids. The interaction with cholesterol indicated that ionic bonds are not necessary, but the nature of the polar group in the 3 position is very important for binding.

The specificity of the interaction of A_1 basic protein and the specificity of Folch-Lees protein, which together make up 85% of the myelin proteins, are the basis of a model of the molecular architecture of the myelin membrane [cf. 495, 496].

8. Beta-Hydroxybutyrate Dehydrogenase

This mitochondrial enzyme has received attention as a model for the study of lipid-protein interactions, since it is readily isolated and its interaction with lipids demonstrates an absolute specificity for lecithin [210]. Lecithin forms an active complex with the enzyme in the presence of a sulfhydryl compound [497]. When the enzyme is released from the membrane, it readily forms an inactive dimer stabilized by S-S bridges. If the dimer is monomerized by SH reagents, lecithin stabilizes the monomer in the form of an enzyme-lecithin complex. Other phospholipids are inactive.

Fleischer and coworkers have reexamined the binding of lipids and their role with β-hydroxybutyrate dehydrogenase. The enzyme was released from mitochondria by phospholipase A [220] and purified 80-fold [498], and an ordered bi-bi mechanism of reaction was found for both soluble and membrane-bound enzyme (both of which require lecithin) [499]. Replacing mitochondrial phospholipids with purified lecithin when reactivating the soluble enzyme results in tighter binding of NADH and NAD to the enzyme, indicating that the lipid environment of the enzyme in the membrane more closely approximates mitochondrial phospholipids than lecithin alone. It has since been shown that lecithin (or a phospholipid mixture containing lecithin) is actually required for binding NADH to the enzyme [500].

The reconstituted system does not have enzymatic activity identical to that in the mitochondrial membrane, however. The mitochondrial enzyme shows a break in the Arrhenius plot at 18 °C [300], whereas the reconstituted enzyme does not show any break with different lipids tested [501]. Recently, however, Houslay et al. [502], using a lipid replacement method, have found that the enzyme is inactive below the phase transition of the lecithins employed. It was suggested that when the apoenzyme is reactivated with aqueous lipid dispersions, it may interact primarily with the choline headgroups of the lecithin, which is absolutely required for activity, but the apoenzyme cannot penetrate the preformed bilayer. When reactivation ensues by lipid exchange in cholate, efficient hydrophobic interactions are possible between the apoenzyme and the lipid chains. If the apoenzyme interacts with the fatty chains, it is sensitive to the physical state of the lipid, whereas if it does not, it is insensitive to lipid crystallization.

X. GENERAL FEATURES OF THE IN VITRO INTERACTIONS

Lipids and proteins combine, but their mode of interaction depends on the previous history of the components, and on the way in which the interacting surfaces are presented to one another. This is very important to consider always before extrapolations can be made to the natural state of the lipid-protein complexes in the intact membrane.

In theory we may summarize the following three principal situations.

    1. If the protein is confronted with bilayer lipids while in the conformational state in which it is present in the membrane, its hydrophobic residues are already exposed, and its penetration of the lipids will usually be possible by direct hydrophobic interaction, provided that the lipid chains are above their transition temperature so that lateral displacements of lipid chains can accommodate the protein (or in an alternative view, fit in crevices between proteins). Such a state is achieved by solvent delipidation that leaves a protein skeleton from protein-rich membranes. For certain very hydrophobic proteins (e.g. Folch-Lees proteolipid) the same result is achieved by solubilization in hydrophobic media. In the first case, the delipidated protein is stabilized by lateral protein-protein hydrophobic contacts and behaves as an insoluble aggregate, but three-dimensional aggregation is prevented by the fact that the intrinsic proteins are amphipathic. In the second case, the protein may be monomeric and lipid chains on the surface are replaced by the nonpolar solvent.

    2. If the protein is extracted from the membrane in a water-soluble form, this means that its conformation may have changed with loss of amphipathy, and random exposure of hydrophilic groups on the entire surface may have ensued. In such case, rebinding with penetration of the membrane requires an initial ionic attraction, followed by "snapping" of the protein into its "hydrophobic" conformation and then penetration.

    3. In the two cases above, the lipids are preformed as bilayers (or monolayers). A third possibility is that lipids are presented to the protein in disaggregated micellar form, induced by presence of detergent. In such a case, mixing the protein with lipids and removing the detergent will allow membrane formation de novo from solubilized components. This method apparently allows reconstitution of intractable components resistant to the other methods, by allowing a more direct hydrophobic contact of protein and lipid.

ACKNOWLEDGMENTS

I am grateful to all those who have sent me reprints and preprints of their work. I also wish to thank Dr. L. Masotti for valuable help and criticism. Dr. A. Spisni has drawn the original figures.

REFERENCES

1. S. J. Singer, Ann. N.Y. Acad. Sci., 195, 16 (1972).
2. R. A. Capaldi and D. E. Green, FEBS Lett., 25, 205 (1972).
3. D. A. Cadenhead, in Progress in Surface Science, ed. J. F. Danielli, A. C. Riddiford, and M. D. Rosenberg, 3, 169 (1970).
4. F. J. Kézdy, in Membrane Molecular Biology, ed. C. F. Fox and A. D. Keith. Stamford: Sinauer Ass., 1972, p. 123.

5. D. Papahadjopoulos, in Form and Function of Phospholipids, 2d ed., ed. G. B. Ansell, R. M. C. Dawson, and J. N. Hawthorne. Amsterdam: Elsevier, 1973, chap. 7.

6. G. Colacicco, Ann. N.Y. Acad. Sci., 195, 224 (1972).

7. G. Colacicco, Lipids, 5, 636 (1970).

8. A. Goldup, S. Ohki, and J. F. Danielli, in Progress in Surface Science, 3, 193 (1970).

9. T. E. Thompson and F. A. Henn, in Membranes of Mitochondria and Chloroplasts, ed. E. Racker. New York: Van Nostrand Reinhold Co., 1970, p. 1.

10. G. Szabo, in Membrane Molecular Biology, ed. C. F. Fox and A. D. Keith. Stamford: Sinauer Ass., 1972, p. 146.

11. H. T. Tien and A. L. Diana, Chem. Phys. Lipids, 2, 55 (1968).

12. A. Finkelstein and A. Cass, J. Gen. Physiol., 52, 145 (1968).

13. M. Montal, Biochim. Biophys. Acta, 298, 750 (1973).

14. K. B. Blodgett, J. Amer. Chem. Soc., 57, 1007 (1935).

15. I. C. P. Smith and K. W. Butler, in Spin Labelling Theory and Application, ed. L. J. Berliner. New York: Academic Press, 1974, chap. 11.

16. J. Seelig, J. Amer. Chem. Soc., 92, 3381 (1970).

17. Y. K. Levine and M. H. F. Wilkins, Nature New Biol., 230, 69 (1971).

18. K. W. Butler, A. W. Hanson, I. C. P. Smith, and H. Schneider. Can. J. Biochem., 51, 980 (1973).

19. I. C. P. Smith, Chemia, 25, 349 (1971).

20. S. Schreier-Muccillo, K. W. Butler, and I. C. P. Smith, Arch. Biochem. Biophys., 159, 297 (1973).

21. C. Mailer, C. P. S. Taylor, S. Schreier-Muccillo, and I. C. P. Smith, Arch. Biochem. Biophys., 163, 671 (1974).

22. A. D. Bangham, Progr. Biophys. Mol. Biol., 18, 29 (1968).

23. A. D. Bangham, Advan. Lipid Res., 1, 65 (1963).

24. A. D. Bangham, in Mitochondria-Biomembranes (Proceedings of the 8th FEBS Meeting, Vol. 28. Amsterdam: North-Holland Publishing Co., 1972, p. 253.

25. A. D. Bangham, M. M. Standish, and I. C. Watkins, J. Mol. Biol., 13, 238 (1965).

26. D. Papahadjopoulos and N. Miller, Biochim. Biophys. Acta, 135, 624 (1967).

27. C. H. Huang, Biochemistry, 8, 344 (1969).

28. R. D. Kornberg and H. M. McConnell, Biochemistry, 10, 1111 (1971).

29. G. Lenaz, G. Curatola, and L. Masotti, J. Bioenergetics, 7, 233 (1975).

30. G. Lenaz, in Membrane Structure and Mechanisms of Biological Energy Transduction, ed. J. Avery. London: Plenum Press, 1973, p. 455.

31. D. Chapman, Lipids, 4, 251 (1969).

32. V. Luzzati, in Biological Membranes. Physical Fact and Functions, ed. D. Chapman. London: Academic Press, 1968, p. 71.

33. R. M. Williams and D. Chapman, Progr. Chem. Fats and Other Lipids, 11, 3 (1970).

34. M. E. Tourtellotte, in Membrane Molecular Biology, ed. C. F. Fox and A. D. Keith. Stamford: Sinauer Ass., 1972, p. 439.

35. D. Chapman, in Biological Membranes, ed. D. Chapman and D. F. H. Wallach, Vol. 2. London: Academic Press, 1973, p. 91.

36. J. Reinert and J. M. Steim, Science, 168, 1580 (1970).

37. D. Chapman, J. Urbina, and K. M. Keough, J. Biol. Chem., 249, 2512 (1974).

38. A. J. Verkleij, B. De Kruyff, P. H. Ververgaert, J. F. Tocanne and L. L. M. Van Deenen, Biochim. Biophys. Acta, 339, 432 (1974).

39. J. F. Tocanne, P. H. Ververgaert, A. J. Verkleij, and L. L. M. Van Deenen, Chem. Phys. Lipids, 12, 201 (1974).

40. B. R. Cater, D. Chapman, S. M. Hawes, and J. Saville, Biochim. Biophys. Acta, 363, 54 (1974).

41. M. C. Phillips, B. D. Ladbrooke, and D. Chapman, Biochim. Biophys. Acta, 196, 35 (1970).

42. J. F. Blazyk and J. M. Steim, Biochim. Biophys. Acta, 266, 737 (1972).

43. M. C. Phillips, B. D. Ladbrooke, and D. Chapman, Chem. Phys. Lipids, 3, 234 (1969).

44. E. Shechter, L. Lettellier, and T. Gulik-Krzywicki, Eur. J. Biochem., 49, 61 (1974).

45. J. Cain, G. Santillan, and J. K. Blasie, in Membrane Research, ed. C. F. Fox. New York: Academic Press, 1972, p. 3.

46. A. Tardieu, V. Luzzati, and F. C. Reman, J. Mol. Biol., 75, 77 (1973).

47. F. Caron, L. Mateu, P. Rigny, and R. Azerad, J. Mol. Biol., 85, 279 (1974).

48. J. L. Ranck, L. Mateu, D. M. Sadler, A. Tardieu, T. Gulik-Krzywicki, and V. Luzzati, J. Mol. Biol., 85, 249 (1974).

49. T. Gulik-Krzywicki, Biochim. Biophys. Acta, 415, 1 (1975).

50. D. Branton, Ann. Rev. Plant Physiol., 20, 309 (1969).

51. H. P. Zingsheim, Biochim. Biophys. Acta, 265, 339 (1972).

52. E. J. Shimshick and H. M. McConnell, Biochemistry, 12, 2351 (1973).

53. C. W. M. Grant, S. H. W. Wu, and H. M. McConnell, Biochim. Biophys. Acta, 363, 151 (1974).

54. P. H. Ververgaert, A. J. Verkleij, P. F. Elbers, and L. L. M. Van Deenen, Biochim. Biophys. Acta, 311, 320 (1973).

55. P. C. Jost, A. S. Waggoner, and O. H. Griffith, in Structure and Function of Biological Membranes, ed. L. I. Rothfield. New York: Academic Press, 1971, p. 83.

56. I. C. P. Smith, in Biological Applications of Electron Spin Resonance, ed. H. M. Swartz, J. R. Bolton, and D. C. Borg. New York: John Wiley & Sons, 1972, p. 483.

57. A. D. Keith, M. Sharnoff, and G. Cohn, Biochim. Biophys. Acta, 300, 379 (1973).

58. E. J. Shimshick, W. Kleemann, W. L. Hubbell, and H. M. McConnell, J. Supramol. Struct., 1, 285 (1973).
59. A. G. Lee, N. J. M. Birdsall, J. C. Metcalfe, P. A. Toon, and G. B. Warren, Biochemistry, 13, 3699 (1974).
60. D. Kivelson, J. Chem. Phys., 33, 1099 (1960).
61. H. Schindler and J. Seelig, J. Chem. Phys., 61, 2946 (1974).
62. J. Israelachvili, J. Sjösten, L. E. G. Eriksson, M. Ehrström, A. Gräslund, and A. Ehrenberg, Biochim. Biophys. Acta, 382, 125 (1975).
63. J. K. Raison, J. M. Lyons, R. J. Mehlhorn, and A. D. Keith, J. Biol. Chem., 246, 4036 (1971).
64. J. K. Raison and E. J. McMurchie, Biochim. Biophys. Acta, 363, 135 (1974).
65. E. Oldfield, K. M. Keough, and D. Chapman, FEBS Letters, 20, 344 (1972).
66. K. W. Butler, N. H. Tattrie, and I. C. P. Smith, Biochim. Biophys. Acta, 363, 351 (1974).
67. J. Seelig and W. Hasselbach, Eur. J. Biochem., 21, 17 (1971).
68. D. Hegner, U. Schummer, and G. H. Schnepel, Biochim. Biophys. Acta, 307, 452 (1973).
69. P. E. Godici and F. R. Landsberger, Biochemistry, 13, 362 (1974).
70. G. Lenaz, G. Parenti-Castelli, A. M. Sechi, E. Bertoli, and D. E. Griffiths, in Membrane Proteins in Transport and Phosphorylation, ed. G. F. Azzone, M. E. Klingenberg, E. Quagliariello, and N. Siliprandi. Amsterdam: North-Holland Publishing Co., 1974, p. 23.
71. D. A. Cadenhead and F. Müller-Landau, in Protides of the Biological Fluids, 21st Colloquium, ed. H. Peeters. New York: Pergamon Press, 1973, p. 175.
72. M. D. Barratt and P. Laggner, Biochim. Biophys. Acta, 363, 127 (1974).
73. N. Z. Stanacev, L. Stuhne-Sekalec, S. Schreier-Muccillo, and I. C. P. Smith, Can. J. Biochem., 52, 884 (1974).
74. A. D. Keith, A. S. Waggoner, and O. H. Griffith, Proc. Nat. Acad. Sci. U.S., 61, 819 (1968).
75. S. I. Ohnishi and T. Ito, Biochemistry, 13, 881 (1974).
76. T. Ito and S. I. Ohnishi, Biochim. Biophys. Acta, 352, 29 (1974).
77. P. Seeman, Pharmacol. Rev., 24, 583 (1972).
78. D. Chapman and G. Dodd, in Structure and Function of Biological Membranes, ed. L. I. Rothfield. New York: Academic Press, 1971, p. 13.
79. G. K. Radda and J. Vanderkooi, Biochim. Biophys. Acta, 265, 509 (1972).
80. W. Lesslauer, J. E. Cain, and J. K. Blasie, Proc. Nat. Acad. Sci. U.S., 69, 1499 (1972).
81. H. Träuble and P. Overath, Biochim. Biophys. Acta, 307, 491 (1973).
82. A. M. Marinangeli, M. Toschi, M. G. Silvestrini, G. Lenaz, and L. Masotti, in preparation (1975).
83. Y. Hatefi and W. G. Hanstein, Proc. Nat. Acad. Sci. U.S., 62, 1129 (1969).

84. G. Lenaz, in Comparative Biochemistry and Physiology of Transport, ed. L. Bolis, K. Bloch, S. E. Luria, and F. Lynen. Amsterdam: North-Holland Publishing Co., 1974, p. 113.

85. J. Augustin and W. Hasselbach, Eur. J. Biochem., 35, 114 (1973).

86. R. A. Badley, W. G. Martin, and H. Schneider, Biochemistry, 12, 268 (1973).

87. H. J. Pownall, A. S. Hu, and L. C. Smith, Biochemistry, 13, 2828 (1974).

88. D. Papahadjopoulos, K. Jacobson, S. Nir, and T. Isac, Biochim. Biophys. Acta, 311, 330 (1973).

89. U. Cogan, M. Shinitzky, G. Weber, and T. Nishida, Biochemistry, 12, 521 (1973).

90. J. F. Faucon and C. Lussan, Biochim. Biophys. Acta, 307, 459 (1973).

91. H. Träuble and H. Eibl, Proc. Nat. Acad. Sci. U.S., 71, 214 (1974).

92. S. Cheng, J. K. Thomas, and C. F. Kulpa, Biochemistry, 13, 1135 (1974).

93. H. J. Galla and E. Sackmann, Biochim. Biophys. Acta, 339, 103 (1974).

94. A. F. Horwitz, in Membrane Molecular Biology, ed. C. F. Fox and A. D. Keith. Stamford: Sinauer Ass., 1972, p. 164.

95. D. Chapman, Ann. N.Y. Acad. Sci., 195, 179 (1972).

96. S. A. Penkett, A. G. Flook, and D. Chapman, Chem. Phys. Lipids, 2, 273 (1968).

97. C. H. A. Seiter and S. I. Chan, J. Amer. Chem. Soc., 95, 7541 (1973).

98. E. G. Finer, J. Magn. Resonance, 13, 76 (1974).

99. M. P. Sheetz and S. I. Chan, Biochemistry, 11, 4573 (1972).

100. D. Lichtenberg, N. O. Petersen, J. L. Girardet, M. Kainosho, P. A. Kroon, C. H. A. Seiter, G. W. Feigenson and S. I. Chan, Biochim. Biophys. Acta, 382, 10 (1975).

101. J. Seelig and W. Niederberger, J. Amer. Chem. Soc., 96, 2069 (1974).

102. J. Seelig and W. Niederberger, Biochemistry, 13, 1585 (1974).

103. J. Seelig and A. Seelig, Biochem. Biophys. Res. Commun., 57, 406 (1974).

104. A. Seelig and J. Seelig, Biochemistry, 13, 4839 (1974).

105. H. Schindler and J. Seelig, Biochemistry, 14, 2283 (1975).

106. H. M. McConnell, P. Devaux, and C. Scandella, in Membrane Research, ed. C. F. Fox. New York: Academic Press, 1972, p. 27.

107. M. Esfahani, E. M. Barnes, and S. J. Wakil, Proc. Nat. Acad. Sci. U.S., 64, 1057 (1969).

108. J. M. Vanderkooi and J. B. Callis, Biochemistry, 13, 4000 (1974).

109. A. G. Lee, N. J. M. Birdsall, and J. C. Metcalfe, Biochemistry, 12, 1650 (1973).

110. C. W. M. Grant and H. M. McConnell, Proc. Nat. Acad. Sci. U.S., 70, 1238 (1973).

111. R. J. M. Smith and C. Green, FEBS Letters, 42, 108 (1974).

112. B. J. Litman, Biochemistry, 13, 2844 (1974).

113. D. M. Michaelson, A. F. Horwitz, and M. P. Klein, Biochemistry, 13, 2605 (1974).
114. C. H. Huang, J. P. Sipe, S. T. Chow, and R. B. Martin, Proc. Nat. Acad. Sci. U.S., 71, 359 (1974).
115. D. M. Michaelson, A. F. Horwitz, and M. P. Klein, Biochemistry, 12, 2637 (1973).
116. J. N. Israelachvili, Biochim. Biophys. Acta, 323, 659 (1973).
117. M. S. Bretscher, Nature New Biol., 236, 46 (1972).
118. M. S. Bretscher, Science, 181, 612 (1973).
119. S. E. Gordesky and G. V. Marinetti, Biochem. Biophys. Res. Commun., 50, 1027 (1973).
120. A. J. Verkleij, R. F. A. Zwaal, B. Roelofsen, P. Comfurius, D. Kastelijn and L. L. M. Van Deenen, Biochim. Biophys. Acta, 323, 178 (1973).
121. A. Casu, G. Nanni, and V. Pala, Ital. J. Biochem., 17, 301 (1968).
122. A. Casu, G. Nanni, U. M. Marinari, V. Pala, and R. Monacelli, Ital. J. Biochem., 18, 154 (1969).
123. G. Nanni, A. Casu, U. M. Marinari, and F. Baldini, Ital. J. Biochem., 18, 25 (1969).
124. G. Nanni, U. M. Marinari, F. Baldini, M. Ferro and A. Casu, Ital. J. Biochem., 18, 123 (1969).
125. A. Kahlenberg, C. Walker, and K. Rohrlick, Can. J. Biochem., 52, 803 (1974).
126. S. Rottem, M. Hasin, and S. Razin, Biochim. Biophys. Acta, 323, 520 (1973).
127. G. Lenaz, L. Landi, P. Pasquali, and L. Cabrini, Arch. Biochem. Biophys., 167, 744 (1975).
128. G. Lenaz, P. Pasquali, E. Bertoli, A. M. Sechi, G. Parenti-Castelli, and L. Masotti, Biochem. Biophys. Res. Commun., 49, 278 (1972).
129. E. Santiago, P. Perez, N. Lopez-Moratalla, and J. Engui, Rev. Esp. Fisiol., 29, 163 (1973).
130. J. L. Segovia, N. Lopez-Moratalla, and E. Santiago, Rev. Esp. Fisiol., 30, 43 (1974).
131. P. Perez, J. Eugui, N. Lopez-Moratalla, J. L. Segovia, and E. Santiago, Rev. Esp. Fisiol., 30, 37 (1974).
132. P. Perez, N. Lopez-Moratalla, and E. Santiago, Rev. Esp. Fisiol., 29, 239 (1973).
133. S. Rottem, Biochem. Biophys. Res. Commun., 64, 7 (1975).
134. B. J. Wisnieski, J. G. Parkes, Y. O. Huang, and C. F. Fox, Proc. Nat. Acad. Sci. U.S., 71, 4381 (1974).
135. W. Renooij, L. M. G. Van Golde, R. F. A. Zwaal, B. Roelofsen, and L. L. M. Van Deenen, Biochim. Biophys. Acta, 363, 289 (1974).
136. C. F. Reed, J. Clin. Invest., 47, 749 (1968).
137. D. Chapman, in Form and Function of Phospholipids, 2nd ed., ed. G. B. Ansell, R. M. C. Dawson, and J. N. Hawthorne. Amsterdam: Elsevier, 1973, chap. 6.

138. B. De Kruyff, R. A. Demel, A. J. Slotboom, L. L. M. Van Deenen, and A. F. Rosenthal, Biochim. Biophys. Acta, 307, 1 (1973).

139. L. L. M. Van Deenen, V. M. T. Houtsmiller, G. H. De Haas, and E. Mulder, J. Pharm. Pharmacol., 14, 429 (1962).

140. D. Chapman and D. F. H. Wallach, in Biological Membranes: Physical Fact and Functions, ed. D. Chapman. New York: Academic Press, 1968, p. 125.

141. D. Ghosh, M. A. Williams, and J. Tinoco, Biochim. Biophys. Acta, 291, 351 (1973).

142. B. De Kruyff, P. W. M. Van Dijck, R. A. Demel, A. Schuijff, F. Brants, and L. L. M. Van Deenen, Biochim. Biophys. Acta, 356, 1 (1974).

143. M. C. Phillips and E. G. Finer, Biochim. Biophys. Acta, 356, 199 (1974).

144. D. Marsh and I. C. P. Smith, Biochim. Biophys. Acta, 298, 133 (1973).

145. S. Schreier-Muccillo, D. Marsh, H. Dugas, H. Schneider, and I. C. P. Smith, Chem. Phys. Lipids, 10, 11 (1973).

146. D. Marsh, Biochim. Biophys. Acta, 363, 373 (1974).

147. R. P. Rand and W. A. Pangborn, Biochim. Biophys. Acta, 318, 299 (1973).

148. M. P. N. Gent and J. N. Prestegard, Biochemistry, 13, 4027 (1974).

149. E. Oldfield and D. Chapman, FEBS Letters, 16, 102 (1971).

150. E. Oldfield and D. Chapman, FEBS Letters, 23, 285 (1972).

151. B. De Kruyff, P. W. M. Van Dijck, R. W. Goldbach, R. A. Demel, and L. L. M. Van Deenen, Biochim. Biophys. Acta, 330, 269 (1973).

152. B. D. Ladbrooke, R. M. Williams, and D. Chapman, Biochim. Biophys. Acta, 150, 333 (1968).

153. J. L. Lippert and W. L. Peticolas, Proc. Nat. Acad. Sci. U.S., 68, 1572 (1971).

154. J. E. Rothman and D. M. Engelman, Nature New Biol., 237, 42 (1972).

155. R. D. Lapper, S. J. Peterson, and I. C. P. Smith, Can. J. Biochem., 50, 969 (1972).

156. D. Marsh and I. C. P. Smith, Biochem. Biophys. Res. Commun., 49, 916 (1972).

157. A. Darke, E. G. Finer, A. G. Flook, and M. C. Phillips, J. Mol. Biol., 63, 265 (1972).

158. K. M. Keough, E. Oldfield, D. Chapman, and P. Beynon, Chem. Phys. Lipids, 10, 37 (1973).

159. W. L. Hubbell and H. M. McConnell, J. Amer. Chem. Soc., 93, 314 (1971).

160. E. Oldfield and D. Chapman, Biochem. Biophys. Res. Commun., 43, 610 (1971).

161. D. L. D. Caspar and D. A. Kirschner, Nature New Biol., 321, 46 (1971).

162. D. Papahadjopoulos, J. Theor. Biol., 43, 329 (1974).

163. B. De Kruyff, R. A. Demel and L. L. M. Van Deenen, Biochim. Biophys. Acta, 255, 331 (1972).
164. J. De Gier, C. W. M. Haest, J. G. Mandersloot, and L. L. M. Van Deenen, Biochim. Biophys. Acta, 211, 373 (1970).
165. D. Papahadjopoulos, M. Cowdon, and H. Kimelberg, Biochim. Biophys. Acta, 330, 8 (1973).
166. S. Fleischer, B. Fleischer, and W. Stoeckenius, J. Cell Biol., 32, 193 (1967).
167. S. Fleischer, G. P. Brierley, H. Klouwen, and D. B. Slautterback, J. Biol. Chem., 237, 3264 (1962).
168. R. S. Criddle, R. M. Bock, D. E. Green, and H. Tisdale, Biochemistry, 1, 827 (1962).
169. D. E. Green and S. Fleischer, Biochim. Biophys. Acta, 70, 554 (1963).
170. G. Schatz and J. Saltzgaber, Biochim. Biophys. Acta, 180, 186 (1969).
171. A. E. Senior and D. H. MacLennan, J. Biol. Chem., 245, 5086 (1970).
172. G. Lenaz, G. Parenti-Castelli, A. M. Sechi, and L. Masotti, Arch. Biochem. Biophys., 148, 391 (1972).
173. G. Lenaz, A. M. Sechi, L. Masotti, and G. Parenti-Castelli, Arch. Biochem. Biophys., 141, 79 (1970).
174. G. Lenaz, A. M. Sechi, G. Parenti-Castelli, and L. Masotti, Arch. Biochem. Biophys., 141, 89 (1970).
175. G. Lenaz. A. M. Sechi, L. Masotti, and G. Parenti-Castelli, Biochem. Biophys. Res. Commun., 34, 392 (1969).
176. T. Olivecrona and L. Oreland, Biochemistry, 10, 332 (1971).
177. R. W. Hendler, Physiol. Rev., 51, 66 (1971).
178. R. F. A. Zwaal and L. L. M. Van Deenen, Chem. Phys. Lipids, 4, 311 (1970).
179. R. F. A. Zwaal and L. L. M. Van Deenen, Biochem. J., 122, 628 (1971).
180. V. B. Kamat, D. Chapman, R. F. A. Zwaal, and L. L. M. Van Deenen, Chem. Phys. Lipids, 4, 323 (1970).
181. P. D. Morse, J. Supramol. Structure, 2, 60 (1974).
182. G. Lenaz, Acta Vitaminol. Enzymol., 27, 62 (1973).
183. P. Zahler and E. R. Weibel, Biochim. Biophys. Acta, 219, 320 (1970).
184. R. Kramer, C. Schlatter, and P. Zahler, Biochim. Biophys. Acta, 282, 146 (1972).
185. P. Schubert, J. Poenzgen, and G. Warner, Hoppe Seyler's Z. Physiol. Chemie, 353, 1034 (1972).
186. V. R. L. Juliano, Biochim. Biophys. Acta, 300, 341 (1973).
187. A. H. Maddy, C. Huang, and T. E. Thompson, Fed. Proc., 25, 933 (1966).
188. R. J. Cherry, K. U. Berger, and D. Chapman, Biochem. Biophys. Res. Commun., 44, 644 (1971).
189. O. Lossen, R. Brennecke, and D. Schubert, Biochim. Biophys. Acta, 330, 132 (1973).

190. D. E. Green and A. Tzagoloff, Arch. Biochem. Biophys., 116, 293 (1966).
191. D. E. Green and A. Tzagoloff, J. Lipid Res., 7, 587 (1966).
192. J. C. Metcalfe, S. M. Metcalfe, and D. M. Engelman, Biochim. Biophys. Acta, 241, 412 (1971).
193. T. Butler, G. L. Smith and E. Grula, Can. J. Microbiol., 13, 1471 (1967).
194. Y. C. Awasthi, T. F. Chuang, T. W. Keenan, and F. L. Crane, Biochim. Biophys. Acta, 226, 42 (1971).
195. G. Vanderkooi, Biochim. Biophys. Acta, 344, 307 (1974).
196. A. K. Parpart and R. Ballentine, in Modern Trends of Physiology and Biochemistry, ed. E. S. G. Barron. New York: Academic Press, 1952, p. 135.
197. B. Roelofsen, J. de Gier, and L. L. M. Van Deenen, J. Cell. Comp. Physiol., 63, 233 (1964).
198. M. T. Sauner and M. Lévy, Biochim. Biophys. Acta, 241, 97 (1971).
199. G. Lenaz, G. Curatola, G. Parenti-Castelli, A. M. Sechi, and E. Bertoli, Abstracts XI Jornadas Bioquimicas Latinas, Salamanca, Spain, 1973.
200. C. Gitler and M. Montal, FEBS Letters, 28, 329 (1972).
201. C. Gitler and M. Montal, Biochem. Biophys. Res. Commun., 47, 1486 (1972).
202. A. A. Benson, J. Amer. Oil Chem. Soc., 43, 265 (1966).
203. G. Vanderkooi, in Protides of the Biological Fluids, ed. H. Peeters. Oxford: Pergamon Press, 1973, p. 157.
204. E. Tria and O. Barnabei, in Structural and Functional Aspects of Lipoproteins in Living Systems, ed. E. Tria and A. M. Scanu. New York: Academic Press, 1969, p. 143.
205. G. P. Brierley, A. Merola, and S. Fleischer, Biochim. Biophys. Acta, 64, 218 (1962).
206. A. Tzagoloff and D. H. MacLennan, Biochim. Biophys. Acta, 92, 476 (1965).
207. L. Rothfield and D. Romeo, in Structure and Function of Biological Membranes, ed. L. I. Rothfield. New York: Academic Press, 1971, p. 251.
208. D. J. Triggle, Progress Surface Science, 3, 273 (1970).
209. R. Tanaka and T. Sakamoto, Biochim. Biophys. Acta, 193, 384 (1969).
210. P. Jurtshuk, I. Sekuzu, and D. E. Green, Biochem. Biophys. Res. Commun., 6, 76 (1961).
211. S. M. Duttera, W. L. Byrne, and M. C. Ganoza, J. Biol. Chem., 243, 2216 (1968).
212. E. Racker, in Membrane Research, ed. C. F. Fox. New York: Academic Press, 1972, p. 97.
213. E. Racker and A. Kandrach, J. Biol. Chem., 248, 5841 (1973).
214. Y. Kagawa and E. Racker, J. Biol. Chem., 246, 5477 (1971).
215. C. I. Ragan and E. Racker, J. Biol. Chem., 248, 6876 (1973).

216. F. Dabbeni-Sala, R. Furlan, A. Pitotti, and A. Bruni, Biochim. Biophys. Acta, 347, 77 (1974).
217. A. D. McLaren and L. Packer, Advan. Enzymol., 33, 245 (1970).
218. E. Katchalski, I. Silman, and R. Goldman, Advan. Enzymol., 34, 445 (1971).
219. Y. C. Awasthi, F. J. Ruzicka, and F. L. Crane, Biochim. Biophys. Acta, 203, 233 (1970).
220. B. Fleischer, A. Casu, and S. Fleischer, Biochem. Biophys. Commun., 24, 189 (1966).
221. S. Estrada, A. T. Carabez, and A. G. Cabeza, Biochemistry, 5, 3432 (1966).
222. P. A. Craven and R. E. Basford, Biochim. Biophys. Acta, 255, 620 (1972).
223. J. D. Jamieson and G. E. Palade, J. Cell Biol., 34, 597 (1967).
224. M. G. Farquhar, in Lysosomes in Biology and Pathology, Vol. 2, ed. J. T. Dingle and H. B. Fell. Amsterdam: North-Holland Publishing Co., 1969, p. 462.
225. J. A. Lucy, in Lysosomes in Biology and Pathology, Vol. 2, ed. J. T. Dingle and H. B. Fell. Amsterdam: North-Holland Publishing Co., 1969, p. 313.
226. G. Sessa and G. Weissmann, J. Biol. Chem., 245, 3295 (1970).
227. L. L. M. Van Deenen, Fed. Proc., 30, 1032 (1971).
228. P. Mitchell, FEBS Letters, 43, 189 (1974).
229. E. Racker and W. Stoeckenius, J. Biol. Chem., 249, 662 (1974).
230. Y. Hatefi, Advan. Enzymol., 25, 275 (1963).
231. D. E. Green, in Comprehensive Biochemistry, Vol. 4, ed. M. Florkin and E. H. Stotz. Amsterdam: Elsevier, 1966, p. 309.
232. A. Kröger and M. Klingenberg, Vit. and Horm., 28, 533 (1970).
233. D. E. Green and I. Silman, Ann. Rev. Plant Physiol., 18, 147 (1967).
234. H. Sandermann, Eur. J. Biochem., 43, 415 (1974).
235. L. I. Rothfield and B. L. Horecker, Proc. Nat. Acad. Sci. U.S., 52, 939 (1964).
236. L. I. Rothfield, M. Takeshita, M. Pearlman, and R. W. Horne, Fed. Proc., 25, 1495 (1966).
237. L. I. Rothfield, 22nd Mosbach Coll. The Dynamic Structure of Cell Membranes. Springer-Verlag, 1971, p. 166.
238. L. I. Rothfield and A. Hinckley, in Comparative Biochemistry and Physiology of Transport, ed. L. Bolis, K. Bloch, S. E. Luria, F. Lynen. Amsterdam: North-Holland Publishing Co., 1974, p. 102.
239. D. Romeo, A. Girard, and L. I. Rothfield, J. Mol. Biol., 53, 475 (1970).
240. D. Romeo, A. Hinckley, and L. I. Rothfield, J. Mol. Biol, 53, 491 (1970).
241. R. M. C. Dawson, in Biological Membranes: Physical Fact and Functions, ed. D. Chapman. London: Academic Press, 1968, p. 203.

242. W. A. Pieterson, J. C. Vidal, J. J. Volwerk, and G. H. de Haas, Biochemistry, 13, 1455 (1974).

243. R. Verger, M. C. E. Mieras, and G. H. de Haas, J. Biol. Chem., 248, 4023 (1973).

244. J. A. F. Op Den Kamp, J. De Gier, and L. L. M. Van Deenen, Biochim. Biophys. Acta, 345, 253 (1974).

245. M. A. Wells, Biochemistry, 13, 2248 (1974).

246. R. M. C. Dawson, in Form and Function of Phospholipids, 2nd ed., ed. G. B. Ansell, R. M. C. Dawson, and J. N. Hawthorne. Amsterdam: Elsevier, 1973, Chapter 5.

247. B. Fourcans and K. M. Jain, Advan. Lipid Res., 12, 147 (1974).

248. J. F. Soodsma and R. Nordlie, Biochim. Biophys. Acta, 191, 636 (1969).

249. W. J. Arion and B. K. Wallin, J. Biol. Chem., 248, 2372 (1973).

250. H. R. Knuell, W. F. Taylor and W. W. Wells, J. Biol. Chem., 248, 5414 (1973).

251. B. Robaire and G. Kato, FEBS Letters, 38, 83 (1973).

252. C. C. Cunningham and L. P. Hager, J. Biol. Chem., 246, 1575 (1971).

253. C. C. Cunningham and L. P. Hager, J. Biol. Chem., 246, 1583 (1971).

254. D. Zakim, J. Biol. Chem., 245, 4953 (1970).

255. D. A. Vessey and D. Zakim, J. Biol. Chem., 246, 4649 (1971).

256. L. Yu, C. Yu, and T. E. King, Biochemistry, 12, 540 (1973).

257. W. L. Zahler and S. Fleischer, J. Bioenergetics, 2, 209 (1971).

258. P. Swanljung, L. Frigeri, K. Ohlson, and L. Ernster, Biochim. Biophys. Acta, 305, 519 (1973).

259. R. Tanaka, T. Sakamoto, and Y. Sakamoto, J. Membrane Biol., 4, 42 (1971).

260. C. Hegyvary, Biochim. Biophys. Acta, 311, 272 (1973).

261. I. C. Cho and H. Swaingood, Biochim. Biophys. Acta, 334, 243 (1974).

262. G. H. Dodd, Eur. J. Biochem., 33, 418 (1973).

263. S. S. Goldman and R. W. Albers, J. Biol. Chem., 248, 867 (1973).

264. A. Martonosi, J. Biol. Chem., 244, 613 (1969).

265. G. Meissner and S. Fleischer, Biochim. Biophys. Acta, 255, 19 (1972).

266. G. S. Levey, Rec. Progr. Hormone Res., 29, 361 (1973).

267. A. Réthy, V. Tomasi, A. Trevisani, and O. Barnabei, Biochim. Biophys. Acta, 290, 58 (1972).

268. P. L. Pedersen, Bioenergetics, 6, 243 (1975).

269. A. E. Senior, Biochim. Biophys. Acta, 301, 249 (1973).

270. R. A. Capaldi, Biochem. Biophys. Res. Commun., 53, 1331 (1973).

271. M. E. Pullman, H. S. Penefsky, A. Datta, and E. Racker, J. Biol. Chem., 235, 3322 (1960).

272. D. H. MacLennan and J. Asai, Biochem. Biophys. Res. Commun., 33, 441 (1968).

273. L. Ernster, K. Nordenbrand, O. Chude, and K. Juntti, in Membrane Proteins in Transport and Phosphorylation, ed. G. F. Azzone, M.

Klingenberg, E. Quagliariello, and N. Siliprandi. Amsterdam: North-Holland Publishing Co., 1974, p. 29.

274. A. Tzagoloff and P. Meagher, J. Biol. Chem., 247, 594 (1972).

275. M. E. Pullman and G. C. Monroy, J. Biol. Chem., 238, 3762 (1963).

276. B. Bulos and E. Racker, J. Biol. Chem., 243, 3891 (1968).

277. B. Bulos and E. Racker, J. Biol. Chem., 243, 3901 (1968).

278. K. J. Cattell, C. R. Lindop, I. G. Knight, and R. B. Beechey, Biochem. J., 125, 169 (1971).

279. F. S. Stekhoven, R. F. Waitkus, and H. T. B. Van Moerkerk, Biochemistry, 11, 1144 (1972).

280. P. Palatini and A. Bruni, Biochem. Biophys. Res. Commun., 40, 186 (1970).

281. J. M. Fessenden-Raden and E. Racker, in Structure and Function of Biological Membranes, ed. L. I. Rothfield. New York: Academic Press, 1971, p. 401.

282. G. Lenaz, G. Parenti-Castelli, and A. M. Sechi, Arch. Biochem. Biophys., 167, 72 (1975).

283. G. Lenaz, G. Parenti-Castelli, A. M. Sechi, E. Bertoli, and D. E. Griffiths, in Membrane Proteins in Transport and Phosphorylation, ed. G. F. Azzone, M. Klingenberg, E. Quagliariello, and N. Siliprandi. Amsterdam: North-Holland Publishing Co., 1974, p. 23.

284. J. M. Broughall, C. R. Lindop, D. E. Griffiths, and R. B. Beechey, Biochem. Soc. Trans., 1, 90 (1972).

285. A. Azzi, C. Montecucco, and M. Santato, in Membrane Proteins in Transport and Phosphorylation, ed. G. F. Azzone, M. Klingenberg, E. Quagliariello, and N. Siliprandi. Amsterdam: North-Holland Publishing Co., 1974, p. 205.

286. A. L. Goldemberg, R. N. Farías, and R. E. Trucco, J. Biol. Chem., 247, 4299 (1972).

287. A. L. Goldemberg, R. N. Farías, and R. E. Trucco, Biochim. Biophys. Acta, 291, 489 (1973).

288. B. Bloj, R. D. Morero, R. N. Farías, and R. E. Trucco, Biochim. Biophys. Acta, 311, 67 (1973).

289. H. Moreno, F. Siñeriz, and R. N. Farías, J. Biol. Chem., 249, 7701 (1974).

290. B. Bloj R. D. Morero, and R. N. Farías, FEBS Letters, 38, 101 (1973).

291. E. M. Massa, R. D. Morero, B. Bloj, and R. N. Farías, Biochem. Biophys. Res. Commun., 66, 115 (1975).

292. F. Siñeriz, R. N. Farías, and R. E. Trucco, FEBS Letters, 32, 30 (1973).

293. F. Siñeriz, B. Bloj, R. N. Farías, and R. E. Trucco, J. Bacteriol., 115, 723 (1973).

294. F. Siñeriz, R. N. Farías, and R. E. Trucco, J. Theor. Biol., 52, 113 (1975).

295. J. K. Raison, in Membrane Structure and Mechanisms of Biological Energy Transduction, ed. J. Avery. London: Plenum Press, 1973, p. 559.

296. A. M. Sechi, L. Landi, E. Bertoli, G. Parenti-Castelli, G. Lenaz, and G. Curatola, Acta Vitamin. Enzymol., 27, 177 (1973).

297. J. Kumamoto, J. K. Raison, and J. M. Lyons, J. Theor. Biol., 31, 47 (1971).

298. V. Massey, B. Curti, and H. Ganther, J. Biol. Chem., 241, 2347 (1966).

299. M. P. Lee and A. R. L. Gear, J. Biol. Chem., 249, 7541 (1974).

300. G. Lenaz, A. M. Sechi, G. Parenti-Castelli, L. Landi, and E. Bertoli, Biochem. Biophys. Res. Commun., 49, 536 (1972).

301. H. K. Kimelberg and D. Papahadjopoulos, J. Biol. Chem., 249, 1071 (1974).

302. S. Rottem, V. P. Cirillo, B. De Kruyff, M. Shinitzky, and S. Razin, Biochim. Biophys. Acta, 323, 509 (1973).

303. G. Inesi, M. Millman, and S. Eletr, J. Mol. Biol., 81, 483 (1973).

304. M. Esfahani, A. R. Limbrick, S. Knutton, T. Oka, and S. J. Wakil, Proc. Nat. Acad. Sci. U.S., 68, 3180 (1971).

305. C. F. Fox and N. Tsukagoshi, Membrane Research, ed. C. F. Fox. New York: Academic Press, 1972, p. 145.

306. B. Bloj, R. D. Morero, and R. N. Farías, J. Nutrition, 104, 1265 (1974).

307. C. D. Linden, A. D. Keith, and C. F. Fox, J. Supramol. Structure, 1, 523 (1973).

308. C. D. Linden, K. L. Wright, H. M. McConnell, and C. F. Fox, Proc. Nat. Acad. Sci. U.S., 70, 2271 (1973).

309. G. B. Warren, N. J. M. Birdsall, A. G. Lee, and J. C. Metcalfe, in Membrane Proteins in Transport and Phosphorylation, ed. G. F. Azzone, M. E. Klingenberg, E. Quagliariello and N. Siliprandi. Amsterdam: North-Holland Publishing Co., 1974, p. 1.

310. R. D. Mavis and P. R. Vagelos, J. Biol. Chem., 247, 652 (1972).

311. S. J. Singer, in Structure and Function of Biological Membranes, ed. L. I. Rothfield. New York: Academic Press, 1971, p. 145.

312. D. W. Urry, Biochim. Biophys. Acta, 265, 115 (1972).

313. D. W. Sears and S. Beychok, in Physical Principles and Techniques of Protein Chemistry. New York: Academic Press, 1973, p. 445.

314. A. J. Adler, N. J. Greenfield and G. D. Fasman, Methods Enzymol., 27, 675 (1973).

315. G. Holzwarth, in Membrane Molecular Biology, ed. C. F. Fox and A. D. Keith. Stamford: Sinauer Ass., 1972, p. 228.

316. D. W. Urry, Methods Enzymol., 32, 220 (1974).

317. D. W. Urry and T. H. Ji, Arch. Biochem. Biophys., 128, 802 (1968).

318. D. W. Urry, J. H. Hinners, and L. Masotti, Arch. Biochem. Biophys., 137, 214 (1970).

319. D. W. Urry, L. Masotti, and J. R. Krivacic, Biochem. Biophys. Res. Commun., 41, 521 (1970).

320. D. W. Urry and J. R. Krivacic, Proc. Nat. Acad. Sci. U.S., 65, 845 (1970).

321. A. S. Schneider, M. J. J. Schneider, and K. Rosenheck, Proc. Nat. Acad. Sci. U.S., 66, 793 (1970).

322. M. Glaser and S. J. Singer, Biochemistry, 10, 1780 (1971).

323. M. Glaser, B. Zimm, and S. J. Singer, Biochemistry, 10, 1785 (1971).

324. D. J. Gordon and G. Holzwarth, Proc. Nat. Acad. Sci. U.S., 68, 2365 (1971).

325. D. W. Urry, L. Masotti, and J. R. Krivacic, Biochim. Biophys. Acta, 241, 600 (1971).

326. L. Masotti, D. W. Urry, J. R. Krivacic, and M. M. Long, Biochim. Biophys. Acta, 266, 7 (1972).

327. D. W. Urry and M. M. Long, in Methods in Membrane Biology, Vol. 1, ed. E. D. Korn. New York: Plenum Press, 1975, p. 105.

328. N. J. Greenfield and G. D. Fasman, Biochemistry, 8, 4108 (1969).

329. D. F. H. Wallach and P. H. Zahler, Proc. Nat. Acad. Sci. U.S., 56, 1552 (1966).

330. J. M. Graham and D. F. H. Wallach, Biochim. Biophys. Acta, 193, 225 (1969).

331. J. M. Graham and D. F. H. Wallach, Biochim. Biophys. Acta, 241, 180 (1971).

332. D. F. H. Wallach, J. M. Graham, and V. R. Fernbach, Arch. Biochem. Biophys., 131, 322 (1969).

333. A. Azzi, B. Chance, G. K. Radda, and C. P. Lee, Proc. Nat. Acad. Sci. U.S., 62, 612 (1969).

334. J. D. Robertson, Biochem. Soc. Symp., 16, 3 (1959).

335. P. Pasquali, L. Landi, L. Masotti, and G. Lenaz, J. Supramol. Structure, 1, 194 (1973).

336. A. S. Gordon, D. F. H. Wallach, and J. H. Strauss, Biochim. Biophys. Acta, 183, 405 (1969).

337. J. Lenard and S. J. Singer, Proc. Nat. Acad. Sci. U.S., 86, 1828 (1966).

338. L. Masotti, D. W. Urry, and R. Llinas, Acta Vitamin. Enzymol., 27, 154 (1973).

339. D. D. Ulmer, B. L. Vallee, A. Gorchein, and A. Neuberger, Nature, 206, 825 (1965).

340. T. Gulik-Krzywicki, E. Shechter, V. Luzzati, and M. Faure, Nature, 223, 1116 (1969).

341. L. Letellier and E. Shechter, Eur. J. Biochem., 40, 507 (1973).

342. K. M. Ivanevitch, J. J. Henderson, and L. S. Kaminsky, Biochemistry, 13, 1469 (1974).

343. A. M. Scanu, Proc. Nat. Acad. Sci. U.S., 54, 1699 (1965).

344. A. M. Gotto and B. Shore, Nature, 224, 69 (1969).

345. S. E. Lux, R. Hirz, R. I. Shrager, and A. M. Gotto, J. Biol. Chem., 247, 2598 (1972).

346. A. M. Scanu and R. Hirz, Proc. Nat. Acad. Sci. U.S., 59, 890 (1968).

347. A. M. Scanu, Biochim. Biophys. Acta, 181, 268 (1969).

348. R. Hirz and A. M. Scanu, Biochim. Biophys. Acta, 207, 364 (1970).

349. R. L. Jackson, A. M. Gotto, S. E. Lux, K. M. John, and S. Fleischer, J. Biol. Chem., 248, 8449 (1973).

350. R. L. Jackson, J. D. Morrisett, H. J. Pownall, and A. M. Gotto, J. Biol. Chem., 248, 5218 (1973).

351. J. D. Morrisett, J. S. K. David, H. J. Pownall, and A. M. Gotto, Biochemistry, 12, 1290 (1973).

352. R. Robson and R. H. Pain, Nature New Biol., 238, 107 (1972).

353. J. Folch-Pi and P. J. Stoffyn, Ann. N.Y. Acad. Sci., 195, 86 (1972).

354. G. Sherman and J. Folch-Pi, J. Neurochem., 17, 597 (1970).

355. Y. London, R. A. Demel, W. S. M. Geurts van Kassel, P. Zahler, and L. L. M. Van Deenen, Biochim. Biophys. Acta, 332, 69 (1974).

356. J. P. Segrest and L. D. Kohn, in Protides of the Biological Fluids, 21st Colloquium, ed. H. Peeters. Oxford: Pergamon, 1973, p. 183.

357. P. M. D. Hardwicke and N. M. Green, Eur. J. Biochem., 42, 183 (1974).

358. J. Lenard and S. J. Singer, Science, 159, 738 (1968).

359. W. L. Zahler, D. Puett, and S. Fleischer, Biochim. Biophys. Acta, 255, 365 (1972).

360. L. Masotti, G. Lenaz, A. Spisni, and D. W. Urry, Biochem. Biophys. Res. Commun., 56, 892 (1974).

361. H. T. Tien and L. K. James, in Chemistry of the Cell Interface, ed. H. D. Brown. New York: Academic Press, 1971, p. 205.

362. R. M. C. Dawson, in Membrane-Bound Enzymes, ed. G. Porcellati and F. Di Jeso. New York: Plenum Press, 1971, p. 1.

363. H. K. Kimelberg and D. Papahadjopoulos, J. Biol. Chem., 246, 1142 (1971).

364. P. J. Quinn and R. M. C. Dawson, Biochem. J., 116, 671 (1970).

365. M. L. Das and F. L. Crane, Biochemistry, 3, 696 (1964).

366. G. G. Shipley, R. B. Leslie, and D. Chapman, Biochim. Biophys. Acta, 173, 1 (1969).

367. G. G. Shipley, R. B. Leslie, and D. Chapman, Nature, 222, 561 (1969).

368. T. Gulik-Krzywicki, E. Shechter, M. Ivatsubo, J. L. Ranck, and V. Luzzati, Biochim. Biophys. Acta, 219, 1 (1970).

369. E. Shechter, T. Gulik-Krzywicki, R. Azerad, and C. Gros, Biochim. Biophys. Acta, 241, 431 (1971).

370. H. K. Kimelberg and D. Papahadjopoulos, Biochim. Biophys. Acta, 233, 805 (1971).

371. A. W. Bernheimer, Biochim. Biophys. Acta, 344, 27 (1974).

372. A. R. Buckelew and G. Colacicco, Biochim. Biophys. Acta, 233, 7 (1971).

373. D. Hegner, U. Schummer, and G. H. Schnepel, Biochim. Biophys. Acta, 291, 15 (1973).
374. S. P. Verma, D. F. H. Wallach, and I. C. P. Smith, Biochim. Biophys. Acta, 345, 129 (1974).
375. M. D. Barratt and L. Rayner, Biochim. Biophys. Acta, 255, 974 (1972)
376. D. O. Shah, Biochim. Biophys. Acta, 193, 217 (1969).
377. C. L. Nicolau, H. Dreeskamp, and D. Schulte-Fröhlinde, FEBS Letters 43, 148 (1974).
378. J. Bello and H. R. Bello, Eur. J. Biochem., 34, 535 (1973).
379. D. Bach and I. R. Miller, J. Membrane Biol., 11, 237 (1973).
380. D. Bach, J. Membrane Biol., 14, 57 (1973).
381. P. T. Shafer, Biochim. Biophys. Acta, 373, 425 (1974).
382. K. Y. Yu, J. J. Baldassare, and C. Ho, Biochemistry, 13, 4375 (1974).
383. C. A. Chang and S. I. Chan, Biochemistry, 13, 4381 (1974).
384. A. Packter and M. Donbrow, Proc. Chem. Soc. London, 220 (1962).
385. G. Prestipino, D. Ceccarelli, F. Conti, and E. Carafoli, FEBS Letters, 45, 99 (1974).
386. P. Calissano, S. Alemà, and P. Fasella, Biochemistry, 13, 4553 (1974).
387. P. Nicholls, Biochim. Biophys. Acta, 346, 261 (1974).
388. K. M. Ivanevitch, J. J. Henderson, and L. S. Kaminsky, Biochemistry, 12, 1822 (1973).
389. P. D. Morse and D. W. Deamer, Biochim. Biophys. Acta, 298, 769 (1973).
390. G. Lenaz, E. Bertoli, L. Landi, G. Parenti-Castelli, P. Pasquali, and A. M. Sechi, in Protides of the Biological Fluids, ed. H. Peeters. Oxford: Pergamon Press, 1973, p. 191.
391. P. Nicholls and A. N. Malviya, Trans. Biochem. Soc., 1, 372 (1973).
392. H. K. Kimelberg, C. P. Lee, A. Claude, and L. Mrena, J. Membrane Biol., 2, 235 (1970).
393. H. K. Kimelberg and C. P. Lee, Biochem. Biophys. Res. Commun., 34, 784 (1969).
394. J. Vanderkooi, M. Erecinska, and B. Chance, Arch. Biochem. Biophys., 154, 219 (1973).
395. G. Parenti-Castelli, E. Bertoli, A. M. Sechi, M. G. Silvestrini, and G. Lenaz, Lipids, 9, 221 (1974).
396. M. L. Das, E. D. Haak and F. L. Crane, Biochemistry, 4, 859 (1965).
397. R. L. Juliano, H. K. Kimelberg, and D. Papahadjopoulos, Biochim. Biophys. Acta, 241, 894 (1971).
398. E. H. Eylar, Ann. N.Y. Acad. Sci., 195, 481 (1972).
399. E. H. Eylar, J. Salk, G. Beveridge, and L. Brown, Arch. Biochem. Biophys., 132, 34 (1969).
400. E. H. Eylar, S. Brostoff, G. Hashim, J. Caccam, and P. Burnett, J. Biol. Chem., 246, 5770 (1971).

401. Y. London and F. G. A. Vossenberg, Biochim. Biophys. Acta, 307, 478 (1973).

402. R. A. Demel, Y. London, W. S. M. Geurts van Kessel, F. G. A. Vossenberg, and L. L. M. Van Deenen, Biochim. Biophys. Acta, 311, 507 (1973).

403. Y. London, R. A. Demel, W. S. M. Geurts van Kessel, F. G. A. Vossenberg, and L. L. M. Van Deenen, Biochim. Biophys. Acta, 311, 520 (1973).

404. J. G. Wood and R. M. C. Dawson, J. Neurochem., 21, 717 (1973).

405. J. G. Wood and R. M. C. Dawson, J. Neurochem., 22, 627 (1974).

406. J. L. Everly, R. O. Brady, and R. H. Quargles, J. Neurochem., 21, 329 (1973).

407. D. Chapman and J. Urbina, FEBS Letters, 12, 169 (1971).

408. E. Bertoli, D. Chapman, S. J. Strach, and D. E. Griffiths, Biochim. Biophys. Acta, submitted (1975).

409. D. Papahadjopoulos, M. Moscarello, E. H. Eylar, and T. Isac, Soc. Trans., 2, 964 (1974).

410. P. Pasquali, E. Bertoli, M. G. Silvestrini, G. Parenti-Castelli, I. Landi, and G. Lenaz, Acta Vitamin. Enzymol., 27, 159 (1973).

411. J. V. Staros and F. M. Richards, Biochemistry, 13, 2721 (1974).

412. J. P. Segrest, T. Gulik-Krzywicki, and C. Sardet, Proc. Nat. Acad. Sci. U.S., 71, 3294 (1974).

413. P. C. Jost, O. H. Griffith, R. A. Capaldi, and G. Vanderkooi, Biochim. Biophys. Acta, 311, 141 (1973).

414. J. Maniloff, G. Vanderkooi, H. Hayashi, and R. A. Capaldi, Biochim. Biophys. Acta, 298, 180 (1973).

415. T. F. Chuang, Y. C. Awasthi, and F. L. Crane, Proc. Indiana Acad. Sci., 79, 110 (1970).

416. P. C. Jost, R. A. Capaldi, G. Vanderkooi, and O. H. Griffith, J. Supramol. Structure, 1, 269 (1973).

417. J. M. Steim, M. E. Tourtellotte, J. C. Reinert, R. N. McElhaney, and R. L. Rader, Proc. Nat. Acad. Sci. U.S., 63, 104 (1969).

418. J. C. Metcalfe, N. J. M. Birdsall, and A. G. Lee, FEBS Letters, 21, 335 (1972).

419. H. M. McConnell, K. L. Wright, and B. G. McFarland, Biochem. Biophys. Res. Commun., 47, 273 (1972).

420. D. M. Engelman, Nature, 223, 1279 (1969).

421. D. M. Engelman, J. Mol. Biol., 58, 153 (1970).

422. D. M. Engelman, Chem. Phys. Lipids, 8, 298 (1972).

423. M. H. F. Wilkins, A. E. Blaurock, and D. M. Engelman, Nature New Biol., 230, 72 (1971).

424. P. Overath, M. Brenner, T. Gulik-Krzywicki, E. Shechter, and L. Letellier, Biochim. Biophys. Acta, 389, 358 (1975).

425. C. W. M. Haest, A. J. Verkleij, J. De Gier, R. Scheek, P. H. J. Ververgaert, and L. L. M. Van Deenen, Biochim. Biophys. Acta, 356, 17 (1974).

426. A. J. Verkleij, P. H. J. Ververgaert, L. L. M. Van Deenen, and P. F. Elbers, Biochim. Biophys. Acta, 288, 326 (1972).
427. R. James and D. Branton, Biochim. Biophys. Acta, 323, 378 (1973).
428. V. Speth and F. Wunderlich, Biochim. Biophys. Acta, 291, 621 (1973).
429. S. Rottem, J. Yashouv, Z. Ne'eman, and S. Razin, Biochim. Biophys. Acta, 323, 495 (1973).
430. P. Pinto da Silva, J. Cell Biol., 53, 777 (1972).
431. G. L. Nicolson, J. Cell Biol., 57, 373 (1973).
432. G. L. Nicolson, J. Supramol. Struct., 1, 410 (1973).
433. T. H. Ji and G. L. Nicolson, Proc. Nat. Acad. Sci. U.S., 71, 2212 (1974).
434. M. Edidin, in Membrane Research, ed. C. F. Fox. New York: Academic Press, 1972, p. 15.
435. W. Junge, FEBS Letters, 25, 109 (1972).
436. P. A. Liebman and G. Entine, Science, 185, 457 (1974).
437. M. Poo and R. A. Cone, J. Supramol. Struct., 1, 354 (1973).
438. M. Poo and R. A. Cone, Nature, 247, 438 (1974).
439. R. Peters, J. Peters, R. H. Tew, and W. Bähr, Biochim. Biophys. Acta, 367, 282 (1972).
440. R. A. Cone, Nature New Biol., 236, 39 (1972).
441. K. Razi-Naqvi, J. Gonzalez-Rodriguez, R. J. Cherry, and D. Chapman, Nature New Biol., 245, 249 (1973).
442. A. S. Kaprelyanz, V. I. Binyukov, D. N. Ostrovskii, G. L. Grigoryan, FEBS Letters, 40, 33 (1974).
443. D. W. Urry, Proc. Nat. Acad. Sci. U.S., 69, 1610 (1972).
444. B. D. Ladbrooke and D. Chapman, Chem. Phys. Lipids, 3, 304 (1969).
445. P. Mueller and D. O. Rudin, Nature, 217, 713 (1968).
446. D. L. Melchior, H. J. Morowitz, J. M. Sturtevant, and T. Y. Tsong, Biochim. Biophys. Acta, 219, 114 (1970).
447. M. E. Tourtellotte, D. Branton, and A. Keith, Proc. Nat. Acad. Sci. U.S., 66, 909 (1970).
448. S. Rottem, W. L. Hubbell, L. Hayflick, and H. M. McConnell, Biochim. Biophys. Acta, 219, 104 (1970).
449. S. Rottem and A. Samuni, Biochim. Biophys. Acta, 298, 32 (1973).
450. Y. Nozawa, H. Iida, H. Fukushima, and K. Ohki, Biochim. Biophys. Acta, 367, 134 (1974).
451. A. F. Esser and J. K. Lanyi, Biochemistry, 12, 1933 (1973).
452. B. M. Sefton and B. J. Gaffney, J. Mol. Biol., 90, 343 (1974).
453. S. Eletr and G. Inesi, Biochim. Biophys. Acta, 290, 178 (1972).
454. F. J. M. Daemen, Biochim. Biophys. Acta, 300, 255 (1973).
455. J. M. P. Borggreven, F. J. Daemen, and S. L. Bonting, Biochim. Biophys. Acta, 202, 374 (1970).
456. N. C. Nielsen, S. Fleischer, and D. G. McConnell, Biochim. Biophys. Acta, 211, 10 (1970).
457. R. E. Anderson and M. B. Maude, Arch. Biochem. Biophys., 151, 270 (1972).

458. S. Futtermann, J. C. Downer, and A. Hendrickson, Invest. Ophthalmol., 10, 151 (1971).

459. J. K. Blasie and C. R. Worthington, J. Mol. Biol., 39, 417 (1969).

460. J. K. Blasie, Biophys. J., 12, 205 (1972).

461. J. K. Blasie, Biophys. J., 12, 191 (1972).

462. R. P. Poincelot, P. Glenn-Millar, R. L. Kimbel, and E. W. Abrahamson, Biochemistry, 9, 1809 (1970).

463. R. E. Anderson and M. B. Maude, Biochemistry, 9, 3625 (1970).

464. J. M. P. Borggreven, J. P. Rotmans, S. L. Bonting, and F. J. M. Daemen, Arch. Biochem. Biophys., 145, 290 (1971).

465. J. M. P. Borggreven, F. J. M. Daemen, and S. L. Bonting, Arch. Biochem. Biophys., 151, 1 (1972).

466. H. Shichi, Exp. Eye Res., 17, 533 (1973).

467. K. Hong and W. L. Hubbell, Proc. Nat. Acad. Sci. U.S., 69, 2617 (1972).

468. M. Zorn and S. Futtermann, J. Biol. Chem., 246, 881 (1971).

469. A. A. Lamola, T. Yamane, and A. Zipp, Biochemistry, 13, 738 (1974).

470. M. L. Applebury, D. M. Zuckerman, A. A. Lamola, and T. M. Jovin, Biochemistry, 13, 3448 (1974).

471. Y. S. Chen and W. L. Hubbell, Exp. Eye Res., 17, 517 (1973).

472. K. Hong, Y. S. Chen, and W. L. Hubbell, J. Supramol. Structure, 1, 355 (1973).

473. M. Montal and J. I. Korenbrot, Nature, 246, 219 (1973).

474. A. Steinemann, C. W. Wu, and L. Stryer, J. Supramol. Structure, 1, 348 (1973).

475. W. E. Wright, P. K. Brown, and G. Wald, J. Gen. Physiol., 62, 509 (1973).

476. F. M. Harold and J. R. Baarda, J. Biol. Chem., 244, 2261 (1969).

477. H. P. Schnebli, A. E. Vatter, and A. Abrams, J. Biol. Chem., 245, 1122 (1970).

478. A. Abrams and C. Baron, Biochemistry, 7, 501 (1968).

479. W. R. Redwood and B. C. Patel, Biochim. Biophys. Acta, 363, 70 (1974).

480. W. R. Redwood and P. Weis, Biochim. Biophys. Acta, 332, 11 (1974).

481. W. R. Redwood, D. C. Gibbes, and T. E. Thompson, Biochim. Biophys. Acta, 318, 10 (1973).

482. S. B. Hladky and D. A. Haydon, Biochim. Biophys. Acta, 274, 294 (1972).

483. P. Strittmatter, J. Biol. Chem., 235, 2492 (1960).

484. L. Spatz and P. Strittmatter, Proc. Nat. Acad. Sci. U.S., 68, 1042 (1971).

485. A. Ito and R. Sato, J. Biol. Chem., 243, 4922 (1968).

486. P. Strittmatter, M. J. Rogers, and L. Spatz, J. Biol. Chem., 247, 7188 (1972).

487. L. Spatz and P. Strittmatter, J. Biol. Chem., 248, 793 (1973).

488. J. Ozols, Biochemistry, 13, 426 (1974).

489. M. J. Rogers and P. Strittmatter, J. Biol. Chem., 249, 895 (1974).

490. P. J. Dehlinger, P. C. Jost, and O. H. Griffith, Proc. Nat. Acad. Sci. U.S., 71, 2280 (1974).

491. M. J. Rogers and P. Strittmatter, J. Biol. Chem., 248, 800 (1973).

492. J. Folch and M. Lees, J. Biol. Chem., 191, 807 (1951).

493. D. S. Chan and M. B. Lees, Biochemistry, 13, 2704 (1974).

494. K. W. Butler, Can. J. Biochem., in press (1975).

495. D. A. Kirschner and D. L. D. Caspar, Ann. N.Y. Acad Sci., 195, 309 (1972).

496. D. L. D. Caspar and D. A. Kirschner, Nature New Biol., 231, 46 (1971).

497. P. Jurtshuk, I. Sekuzu, and D. E. Green, J. Biol. Chem., 238, 3595 (1963).

498. N. C. Nielsen and S. Fleischer, J. Biol. Chem., 248, 2549 (1973).

499. N. C. Nielsen, W. L. Zahler, and S. Fleischer, J. Biol. Chem., 248, 2556 (1973).

500. P. Gazzotti, H. G. Bock, and S. Fleischer, Biochem. Biophys. Res. Commun., 58, 309 (1974).

501. S. Fleischer, H. G. Bock, and P. Gazzotti, in Membrane Proteins in Transport and Phosphorylation, ed. G. F. Azzone, M. E. Klingenberg, E. Quagliariello, and N. Siliprandi. Amsterdam: North-Holland Publishing Co., 1974, p. 125.

502. M. D. Houslay, G. B. Warren, N. J. M. Birdsall, and J. C. Metcalfe, FEBS Letters, 51, 146 (1975).

Chapter 4

THE Ca^{2+}-Mg^{2+} ATPase PROTEIN OF SARCOPLASMIC RETICULUM

Ronald J. Baskin

Department of Zoology
University of California
Davis, California

I. INTRODUCTION

The internal membrane system of striated muscle, the sarcoplasmic reticulum (SR), first described by Veratti [1], is now know to regulate the contraction-relaxation cycle. This system has two, membrane-linked functions: the liberation of Ca^{2+} on excitation and the ATP-mediated accumulation of this Ca^{2+} to a level that allows relaxation [2-4]. Intact sarcoplasmic reticulum consists of a series of membranous tubules and cisternae. During isolation, these structures are fragmented and reseal into a suspension of spherical vesicles (FSR). These vesicles constitute a membrane transport system that can transport calcium in an ATP-dependent reaction.

Extensive transport of calcium has been shown by experiments in which anions such as oxalate or phosphate (both of which are readily permeable) were added to vesicular suspensions before addition of ATP [5, 6]. With either of these anions present, extensive calcium precipitates could be located within the FSR vesicles.

Thus, this system has been used as a model for the study of membranes that carry out energy transduction [6-8]. Its central component is the Ca^{2+}-Mg^{2+} ATPase protein, which makes up the largest proportion of the total of all proteins. This protein is involved in binding and transporting Ca^{2+} and perhaps also in releasing it.

Little is now known about how calcium is released from sarcoplasmic reticulum membranes. Depolarization of the muscle-cell membrane continues along the T-system membranes. At approximately one-sarcomere intervals along a myofibril, the T system intersects regions of the sarcoplasmic reticulum. The junctional properties of these intersecting regions are not understood. Thus the means by which depolarization of the T-system membranes causes the sarcoplasmic reticulum to release Ca^{2+} is not known.

In contrast to the mechanism of Ca^{2+} release, much information has been obtained on the mechanism of Ca^{2+} accumulation. The ATPase protein that is responsible for this accumulation of Ca^{2+} will be discussed in detail. Extensive discussions of earlier work can be found in numerous reviews [9, 10].

II. ISOLATION OF THE Ca^{2+}-Mg^{2+} ATPase PROTEIN

Procedures for isolating fragmented sarcoplasmic reticulum membranes are well developed and are based on the differential centrifugation technique of Portzehl [11] and Lorand et al. [12]. Extracting sarcoplasmic reticulum preparations with 0.6 M KCl followed by centrifuging removes most of the contaminating myosin [13]. Further purification can be accomplished by density-gradient centrifugation in continuous or discontinuous sucrose density gradients [14] or by zonal centrifugation [15]. In spite of these techniques, some contaminating particles and membranes are present in preparations of fragmented sarcoplasmic reticulum. Since some of these membranes contain an ATPase that is not calcium-sensitive, measurement of this ATPase indicates the extent of contamination. Damaged FSR vesicles are not recognized by this technique since they may have an active Ca^{2+}-sensitive ATPase activity but be unable to sequester calcium.

Sarcoplasmic reticulum proteins can be resolved using SDS gel electrophoresis [16, 17]. The major component of the gel is the 100,000- to 106,000-dalton protein (Fig. 1). This protein was shown to be the ATPase, since ^{32}P from ATP-γ-^{32}P was incorporated into it and not into other components of the FSR membranes. Two other proteins of molecular weight 44,000 and 55,000 daltons are present in relatively high concentrations. The higher-molecular-weight protein has been referred to as a high-affinity calcium binding protein and the 44,000-dalton protein has been called calsequestrin [18, 19].

Smaller proteins with a molecular weight in the range 20,000 to 30,000 daltons are also seen. It has recently been suggested that they may be the result of proteolytic digestion of calsequestrin [20]. Finally, a proteolipid

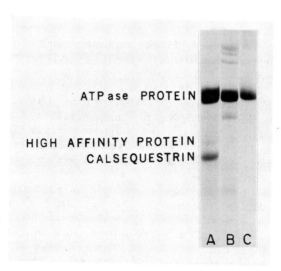

FIG. 1 SDS gels of (A) rabbit SR, (B) lobster SR, and (C) lobster ATPase, prepared by the method of Warren et al. [26]. Arrow indicates Ca^{2+}-Mg^{2+} ATPase protein with a molecular weight of 106,000 daltons. The lower dark band in the rabbit SR preparation is calsequestrin; the faint band above it is the "calcium-binding protein." The lobster SR preparation shows, in addition to the ATPase band, only a faint band at the 85,000-dalton region. The lobster ATPase preparation shows only the 106,000-dalton band.

with a mobility in SDS gels equivalent to a molecular weight of 6,000 has been isolated [21].

Purification of the ATPase protein has been tried by numerous investigators. Martonosi [22] first succeeded in purifying the ATPase enzyme using deoxycholate and salt, although in these experiments a large amount of activity of the enzyme was lost. MacLennan [19] modified the procedure by first removing loosely bound and water-soluble proteins (extrinsic membrane proteins) from a lipid-bound and water-insoluble fraction including the Ca^{2+} ATPase (intrinsic membrane proteins) with low levels of deoxycholate in the presence of 1 M KCl. The intrinsic membrane protein fraction was then dissolved in a higher concentration of deoxycholate and the Ca^{2+} ATPase fractionated by precipitation with ammonium acetate. The ATPase activity finally obtained 28-35 μmole of ATP hydrolyzed per min per mg of protein (37 °C), was increased three times over the value at the start, and retained sensitivity to both calcium and magnesium. Gel electrophoresis indicated that a protein with a molecular weight of about 102,000 daltons accounted for more than 90% of the protein of the purified ATPase. This protein was phosphorylated following the reaction with (λ = ^{32}P) ATP and Ca^{2+}, proving that it contained the active site for ATP hydrolysis. The purified ATPase preparation also contained a proteolipid that had two molecules of fatty acid covalently bonded to a protein molecule of molecular weight 12,000 daltons. The proteolipid in contrast to the ATPase enzyme was not phosphorylated [23]. Its role in the purified ATPase preparation is not currently understood.

Another method for purifying the Ca^{2+}-Mg^{2+} ATPase was developed by Warren et al. [24-26]. This involves treating FSR vesicles with DOC (0.4 mg/mg protein) and centrifugation at 190,000 g. The supernatant solution was layered on a sucrose gradient. When the lipid-protein complexes reached the boundary between the DOC and the sucrose gradient, they broke through, re-formed particulate material, and sedimented to an equilibrium position in the gradient. Low-molecular-weight proteins remained in the detergent layer. The upper part of the main protein peak contained the ATPase protein at a purity of more than 95%.

A significant feature of this procedure is that during sedimentation, 99.7% of the added DOC is removed. The remaining 0.3% corresponds to less than one molecule of DOC per ATPase molecule. In contrast to the MacLennan procedure, only 25%-30% of the original SR lipid is retained in the purified ATPase using this method. There is, however, no evidence for the selective removal of any particular phospholipid class. Neither this preparation nor the MacLennan preparation can accumulate calcium.

Solubilization of FSR membranes in Triton X-100 followed by removal of phospholipid by chromatography on a sepharose column results in the loss of calcium-dependent ATPase activity [27]. Adding phospholipids, fatty acids, or various synthetic lipids results in the restoration of a calcium-independent ATPase activity, but not of calcium-dependent ATPase activity or calcium accumulation.

Partial purification of FSR vesicles has also been accomplished by adding lysolecithin (1 to 2 mg per mg of protein) followed by differential centrifugation [28]. This procedure increases the calcium-sensitive ATPase activity approximately twofold. The Ca^{2+}-Mg^{2+} ATPase makes up 75%–80% of the protein in the purified fraction. Lysolecithin displaces much of the original lipid and represents 65% of the lipid phosphate in the lysolecithin-ATPase complex. SDS gel electrophoresis shows a single large band of about 105,000 daltons. This band is not affected by reduction with β-mercapto-ethanol.

III. AMINO ACID COMPOSITION AND SUBUNITS

The amino acid composition of the Ca^{2+}-Mg^{2+} ATPase protein has been determined independently by numerous investigators [15, 23, 27]. As Table 1 indicates, the various determinations are in good agreement. Acidic

TABLE 1

Amino Acid Composition of the Ca^{2+}-Mg^{2+} ATPase Protein

Amino acid	Moles percent		
	(a)	(b)	(c)
Lysine	5.84	6.47	5.42
Histidine	1.52	1.07	1.27
Arginine	4.76	8.09	5.08
Aspartic acid	9.76	9.67	8.72
Threonine	5.53	6.56	5.90
Serine	5.49	5.41	5.00
Glutamic acid	12.20	14.54	10.60
Proline	5.05	4.78	5.50
Glycine	8.45	4.35	7.03
Alanine	9.80	6.34	8.48
Cysteic acid	2.52	2.78	2.33
Valine	7.55	8.29	7.66
Methionine	1.36	4.09	3.39
Isoleucine	5.60	5.48	6.18
Leucine	9.81	11.96	9.75
Tyrosine	2.15	3.68	2.33
Phenylalanine	3.94	6.29	5.30

Source: Data of Martonosi and Halpin [17] in (a), MacLennan et al. [23] in (b), and Meissner et al. [15] in (c)

TABLE 2

Estimate of Percentage of Total SR Protein Composing
the Ca^{2+}-Mg^{2+} ATPase Protein

Yu and Masoro [29]	"Fraction 2"	90%
McFarland and Inesi [33]	"90,000 dalton"	60%
MacLennan, Ostwald, and Stewart [32]	"ATPase"	35%-45%
Meissner, Conner, and Fleisher [15]	"ATPase"	60%-70%
Deamer [28]	"ATPase"	50%

amino acids (about 20% of the total residues) outnumber the basic amino
acids by two to one. Strongly hydrophilic molecules such as glutamic and
aspartic acids, lysine, and arginine account for about 30% of the total amino
acids.

It was claimed that reducing agents such as β-mercaptoethanol dissociated proteins of FSR into 20,000-60,000-dalton subunits [29, 30]. However,
this has not been confirmed by more recent studies [28, 31]. It appears then
that the Ca^{2+} ATPase is a single polypeptide chain.

Estimates of the percentage of membrane protein that makes up the
Ca^{2+}-Mg^{2+} ATPase protein vary from 35% to 90% (Table 2). The 90% estimate obtained by Yu and Masoro [29] is for a "fraction-2," which may have
contained other proteins in addition to the Ca^{2+}-Mg^{2+} ATPase protein; thus
this estimate is most likely too high. The lowest estimate, 35%-45%, made
by MacLennan et al. [32], may have been made using an initial FSR preparation that contained impurities. If this were the case, then their estimate
would be too low. The estimate Meissner et al. [15] made of 60%-70% was
based on using carefully purified FSR and determining activity referred to
phosphoenzyme production. Furthermore, the authors argue quite convincingly, this is the only reliable method available for the estimating activity.
This method requires, however, assuming a protein molecular weight of
105,000 daltons and the presence of one phosphoenzyme site per molecule.
Estimates by Deamer [28] and McFarland and Inesi [33] are close to the
estimates of Meissner et al. [15]. Thus a figure of 60%-70% of the total FSR
protein as composing the Ca^{2+}-Mg^{2+} ATPase protein appears the best estimate at present.

IV. MEMBRANE ORGANIZATION OF THE Ca^{2+}-Mg^{2+} ATPase PROTEIN

Fragmented sarcoplasmic reticulum (FSR) isolated by differential centrifugation (Fig. 2A) shows generally spherical vesicles [34]. Thin sections of
pelleted preparations show a triple-layered membrane 60-70 Å thick [4].
The appearance is of a typical "unit membrane," as described for most

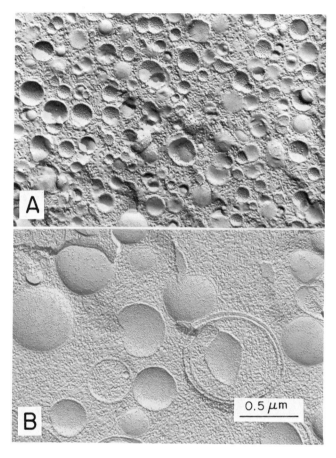

FIG. 2 Freeze-fracture micrographs of (A) sarcoplasmic reticulum vesicles and (B) ATPase vesicles. ATPase vesicles are generally larger and contain particles on both concave and convex fracture faces. SR vesicles have most of the 80-Å particles on the concave fracture face. The total particle density (both concave and convex faces) of each preparation is approximately equal.

biological membranes prepared in this way [35]. Vesicle diameter seems to vary from preparation to preparation and probably depends on handling during preparation. We routinely obtain vesicles from lobster SR in the range 1,800-Å diameter. They range in size from 300 Å to approximately 3,500 Å [36]. The method of thin sectioning does not allow identifying the protein and the lipid portions of the membrane. Agostini and Hasselbach [37], using the electron-dense SH reagent Hg-phenyl azoferritin, have shown that this reagent binds to the exterior membrane surface but not to the interior surface; this finding indicates that FSR membranes are asymmetrically built. The Ca^{2+}-Mg^{2+} ATPase lipoprotein also forms vesicles when the detergent is removed. Thin-sectioned electron micrographs show vesicles identical to those seen in FSR preparations.

Vesicles prepared by negative staining with uranylacetate or phosphotungstate [38] show a characteristically different appearance from those prepared by thin sectioning. Following negative staining, FSR vesicles show the presence of 40-Å-diameter spherical particles covering the vesicle surface [34, 39, 40]. The center-to-center separation of the particles is 90–100 Å. Despite an earlier report to the contrary [23], vesicles formed from the Ca^{2+}-Mg^{2+} ATPase show the presence of 40-Å-diameter particles following negative staining [31, 41].

Trypsin treatment removes the 40-Å surface particle both from FSR vesicles [39] and from ATPase vesicles [31]. Conditions that protect the ATPase activity from the action of trypsin (1 M sucrose, 5 mM ATP) also decrease the ability of trypsin to cause removal of the surface particles. The hypothesis has been presented that these "negative-stain" particles represent a portion of the ATPase molecule [31, 41]. The earlier work of Hasselbach and Elfvin [42], which showed the binding of azoferritin, an agent that binds to SH groups, to structures on the vesicle membrane surface, supports the concept of an active site at the membrane surface but provides no evidence about the structure of the active site or its relation to the 40-Å negative stain particles. Indeed, the results of Ikemoto et al. [43] directly contradict this hypothesis. They concluded that surface "spheres and stalks" affect Ca^{2+} transport little or not at all. Since the negative stain technique involves the air drying of unfixed membranes, the resulting structures must be interpreted with caution. Even so, owing simply to the presence of the ATPase protein in such a large amount relative to any other protein, it is likely that the 40-Å negative-stain particles are related to the presence of this protein. Clearly defined electron micrographs of single ATPase molecules have not yet been obtained. The purified ATPase solubilized in the presence of Triton X-100 or deoxycholate shows mainly amorphous aggregates following negative staining [23, 41].

Freeze-fracturing studies on preparations of FSR vesicles (Fig. 2A) have shown the presence, within the membrane bilayer, of 80-Å particles [34, 44, 45]. Freeze-fracturing has been shown to cleave membranes within the hydrophobic interior and along a plane parallel to the plane of the mem-

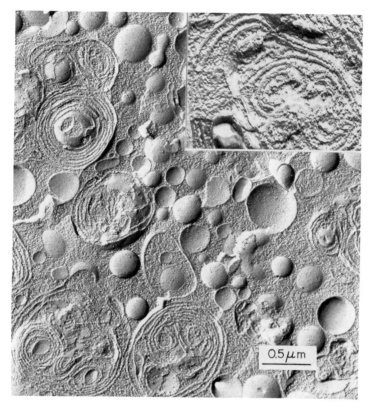

FIG. 3 Freeze-etch micrograph of ATPase vesicles prepared from lobster SR by the method of MacLennan [19]. Some vesicles contain many membrane layers. Individual layers show a low-density region between two dense areas (inset).

brane [46]. The concave freeze-etch face is derived from the outer, or cytoplasmic, portion of the membrane bilayer (Fig. 2). The convex face is derived from the inner, or cisternal, portion. The reason for the absence of complementary fracture faces is not completely understood; the studies of Flower [47], however, strongly indicate that the holes are probably lost in most membrane faces by distortion during fracturing. These membrane particles [23] are also seen in vesicle membranes prepared from the Ca^{2+}-Mg^{2+} ATPase (Fig. 3). This provides strong support for the contention that these particles represent the ATPase protein. Studies of the development of the calcium transport system also support this contention, since the development of the 80-Å particles parallels the development of calcium transport [48, 49].

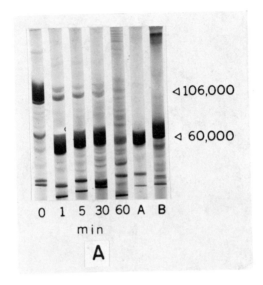

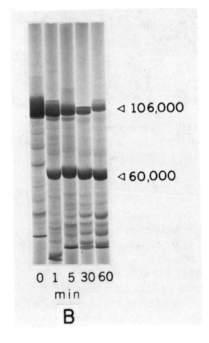

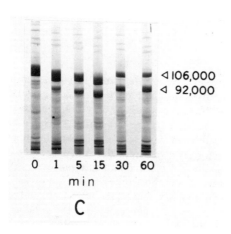

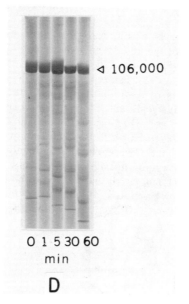

FIG. 4 (Left and above) SDS gels showing the effect of various periods of trypsinization (1% solution) on (A) rabbit SR, (B) rabbit ATPase, (C) lobster SR, and (D) lobster ATPase. While trypsin acts to break the rabbit Ca^{2+}-Mg^{2+} ATPase protein into two fragments of nearly equal size (50,000–60,000 daltons), its action on the lobster Ca^{2+}-Mg^{2+} ATPase protein is different. The trypsin-sensitive region on this protein is apparently located nearer to one end of the polypeptide chain, since a 92,000-dalton fragment and a small (~15,000-dalton) fragment result. Lobster preparations appear more resistant to trypsin than rabbit preparations do, and the ATPase preparation of each more resistant than the SR preparation. The A gel contains catalase (MW = 57,000 daltons) and the B gel bovine serum albumin (MW = 67,000 daltons).

161

Exactly what the 80-Å particles actually represent is not known. Allowing for a 10-20-Å layer of metal shadow, the actual particle size is nearer to 60 Å in diameter. This may represent only the protein moiety or a combination of lipid and protein. (Freeze-fractures of liposomal membranes typically show smooth-surfaced vesicles [R. J. Baskin, unpublished data; 50].

Trypsin has been shown to affect the ATPase activity of FSR vesicles. Sodium dodecyl stearate gel electrophoresis patterns of FSR vesicles subjected to trypsinization show the rapid breakdown of the ATPase protein (from rabbit) into two subfragments [51, 52]. One subfragment has a molecular weight of approximately 60,000 daltons and the other a molecular weight of approximately 55,000 daltons (Fig. 4). Prolonged trypsinization results in the breakdown of the 60,000-dalton subfragment into smaller fragments [31, 51].

Treating FSR vesicles with trypsin for short periods (Fig. 5) did not affect the appearance of the 80-Å freeze-etch particles [31]. Prolonged trypsinization, however, resulted in the clumping of some particles and the extraction of others (Fig. 6). Table 3 indicates the effects of trypsinization on 80-Å particle density in vesicles of FSR and purified ATPase. ATPase membranes appear quite resistant to the action of trypsin. This effect can also be seen in the SDS gels (Fig. 4) of normal and trypsinized membranes.

The 80-Å freeze-fracture particles may be asymmetrically located in the FSR vesicle membrane. Evidence for this location is provided by the observation that the cytoplasmic face of the vesicle (concave face) contains most of the particles (4,000 particles/μ^2) while the cisternal face (convex face) contains only a few particles (500 particles/μ^2) (see Fig. 2A). The situation is entirely different in vesicles obtained from purified Ca^{2+}-Mg^{2+}

TABLE 3

Particle Density of Concave Vesicles
(Particles/μ^2)

	FSR	ATPase
Rabbit (Normal),	3,900	2,476
1% trypsin		
5 min	4,013	
1 hr		2,374
Lobster (Normal),	3,860	2,203
1% trypsin		
1 min	3,584	1,908
30 min	2,240	
3 hr	480[a]	

[a]"Clumped" particles.

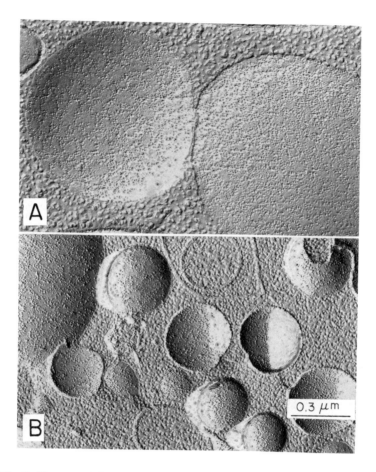

FIG. 5 Freeze-etch micrograph of rabbit ATPase vesicles (A) before and (B) after treatment with 1% trypsin solution for one hour. While the gels indicated (Fig. 4B) that over half the ATPase protein was split into two fragments, the particle density on both concave and convex faces of the vesicles was unchanged. Thus the cleaved protein fragments remained in the original membrane location.

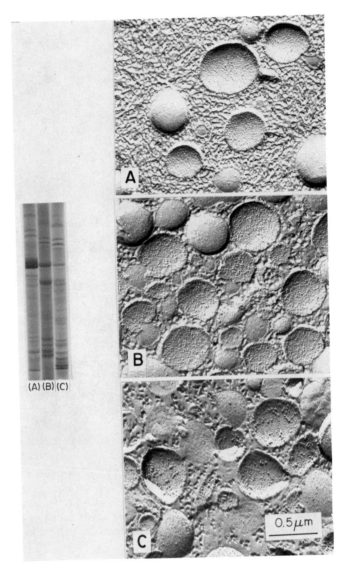

FIG. 6 Freeze-etch micrographs of trypsin treated lobster SR vesicles.
(A) Untreated vesicles are contrasted with vesicles having (B) 30 min and
(C) 180 min of exposure to 1% trypsin. Gels show the extent of fragmentation
at each time. Following 180 min of exposure, a substantial decrease of
particle density on both vesicle faces is observed. The remaining particles
are large, possibly representing clumping of fragments.

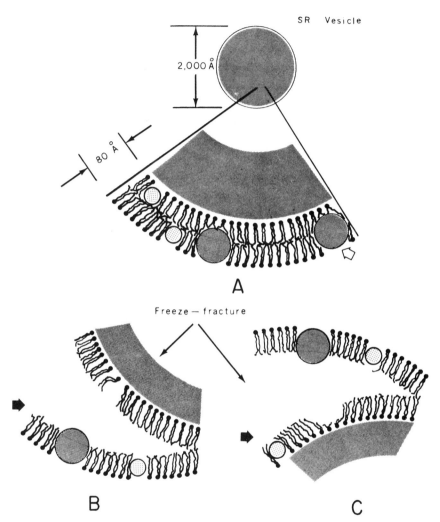

FIG. 7 A. Diagram of the postulated location in the SR membrane of the ATPase protein (open arrow). The basis for the resulting difference in particle density in the (B) concave and (C) convex faces is indicated.

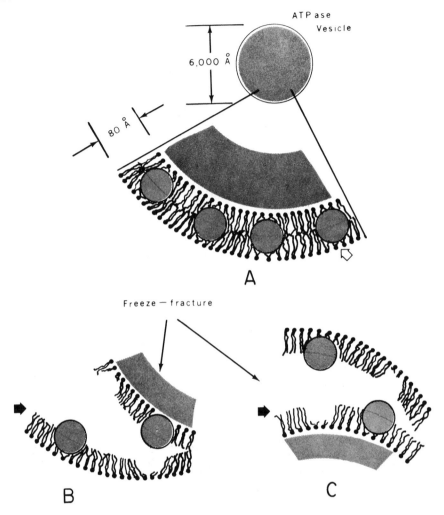

FIG. 8 A. Diagram of the postulated membrane location of the ATPase protein in vesicles formed from the purified ATPase preparation. Due to the symmetrical location, particle densities would be similar on both fracture faces (B and C).

ATPase. In this case (Fig. 2B), the particle density is the same on both faces of the membrane (2,500 particles/μ^2), most likely indicating a symmetrical location within the membrane of the 80-Å particle [53]. The hypothesis relating the relative particle densities to the location in the membrane of the ATPase protein is illustrated in Figures 7 and 8.

It has been speculated [51] that the site of the initial trypsin attack might be the "stalk" of the 40-Å surface particle appearing following negative staining of FSR vesicles or of ATPase vesicles. These particles are not seen by any other technique (i.e., thin sections, freeze-etch), however, even though they do show the vesicle surface. The vesicle "surface" as seen following negative staining represents the compaction of many layers of collapsed membrane, all of which have been subjected to substantial forces during drying. As a consequence of this treatment, alteration of the normal surface structure could occur. Further studies are therefore needed to determine precisely the site of action of trypsin.

An interesting alteration in the density of 80-Å freeze-fracture particles has been observed in FSR vesicles obtained from dystrophic chicken muscle [54, 55]. The density of these particles appears to be substantially lower in the dystrophic vesicles than in the normal. This may be a basic membrane alteration that is characteristic of the disease, but further studies will be necessary to establish this idea firmly, since these preparations contain contaminating membranes as well as SR membranes. It must be shown that the apparent difference in particle density is characteristic of SR membranes and does not result from a difference in the quantity of non-SR membrane present in each of the preparations.

X-ray diffraction studies have been carried out on preparations of packed FSR vesicles [56-59]. While all the investigators find that the electron-density profile of the membrane is asymmetric, there is no agreement about the location of the asymmetric portion. Liu and Worthington [57] argue that the asymmetry is explained by the presence of the ATPase protein in the inner, or cisternal, side of the vesicle membrane, while Dupont et al. [58] consider it to be located in the outer, or cytoplasmic, portion of the membrane. The latter location agrees with the freeze-fracture data, which provide evidence for locating the ATPase molecules (80-Å particles) asymmetrically toward the outer portion of the membrane bilayer.

V. INTERACTION OF THE Ca^{2+}-Mg^{2+} ATPase PROTEIN WITH LIPIDS

The lipid content of both the total FSR membrane and the ATPase purified according to MacLennan's method has been determined [60, 61]. The purified ATPase contains approximately 600 μg lipid per mg protein with 90% phospholipid and 10% neutral lipid (Table 4). Approximately 97% of the neutral lipid is cholesterol. About 66% of the phospholipid is phosphatidylcholine. Phosphatidylethanolamine, phosphatidylinositol, and phosphatidylserine make up

TABLE 4

Lipid Composition of the Purified Ca^{2+}-Mg^{2+} ATPase

	μmole lipid per 100 mg protein
Phosphatidylcholine	40.0
Phosphatidylethanolamine	10.2
Phosphatidylserine	6.85
Sphingomyelin	2.79
Cardiolipin	0.23
Total phospholipid	60.07
Cholesterol	15.3
Triglycerides	0.45
Total neutral lipid	15.75
Total lipid	75.82

Source: Data of MacLennan et al. [23] and Marai and Kuksis [60].
Note: Purified according to the method of MacLennan [19].

most of the remainder. The composition and molecular association of the fatty acids in the phosphatides of FSR and purified ATPase have been examined [61]. Rabbit skeletal muscle was shown to contain fatty acids different from those found in other animals [61]. The triglyceride composition was unusual in the high content of simple triglycerides.

Of particular interest is the part lipids have in the ATPase and calcium-binding and transport activities of the protein. An absolute requirement for phospholipid in these processes has been clearly shown [16, 62, 63]. Three different approaches have been used to study the role of lipids. Lipid depletion of membranes has been achieved by treatment with phospholipases. Solvent extraction of lipids has been used, and also lipid substitution techniques [24, 26, 28, 64].

As used thus far, solvent extraction techniques have the very severe effect of inhibiting the calcium transport and ATPase activities in FSR membranes. They have not been used on the purified ATPase preparation.

Lipid depletion of membranes by using phospholipases has been an important method for analyzing what phospholipids do in calcium transport and ATPase activity. The phospholipases have the advantage of specificity of action and reversible modification of functional properties of membranes.

Phospholipase C is able to cause rapid inhibition of both ATPase activity and calcium transport in FSR vesicles [13, 65]. This is accompanied by extensive hydrolysis of membrane lecithin [66]. The reaction products of this hydrolysis are phosphorylcholine and diglycerides. Their accumulation was not responsible for the effects of phospholipase C on FSR vesicles [67]. It has been reported that there is some restoration of both calcium transport activity and ATPase activity when micellar dispersions of lecithin or lyso-lecithin were added to microsomes treated with phospholipase C [66].

The basis for the inhibition of calcium transport and ATPase activity may be looked on as a requirement for lecithin either in the formation or in the decomposition of the phosphorylated intermediate. Since the maximum steady-state concentration of phosphoprotein is apparently insensitive to phospholipase C, it has been suggested that the inhibition of ATP hydrolysis is related to a lecithin requirement for the hydrolysis of the phosphoprotein intermediate [63, 65]. Evidence has also been presented that indicates that phospholipase C treatment and the subsequent lipid removal reduces the dependence of the formation of the phosphoprotein intermediate on calcium.

Phospholipase C isolated from B. cereus shows effects on FSR vesicles similar to the effects caused by the C. welchii preparation, except that this enzyme is able to hydrolyze phosphatidylcholine, phosphatidylserine, and phosphatidylethanolamine [65]. Phospholipase C (C. welchii) did not attack ethanolamine or serine phospholipids and left 10%-20% of the lecithin unaffected.

FSR vesicles have been treated with phospholipase A (Crotalus terrificus terrificus). This causes the liberation of free fatty acids and lysophosphatides [65, 68]. The detergent effect of the free fatty acids causes an increase in permeability to calcium, inhibits calcium uptake, and activates ATP hydroly-sis without causing any change in the steady-state concentration of phospho-protein. Removing the liberated fatty acids and lysophosphatides by washing with serum albumin [69] resulted in an inhibition of ATPase activity. Adding lysolecithin [65] or lecithin [63] to phospholipase-A-treated FSR vesicles caused some restoration of ATPase activity.

Phospholipase D treatment causes the hydrolysis of the major portion of membrane lecithin in FSR vesicles into phosphatidic acid and choline. This hydrolysis does not result in inhibition of calcium transport or of ATPase activity, most likely because the phosphatidic acid is retained in the mem-brane [66, 68].

Fragmented sarcoplasmic reticulum vesicles have been extracted with a variety of organic solvents, including acetone [13], ether [70, 71], and aqueous heptane [72]. Treating both with acetone and with ether leads to an inhibition of calcium transport. Acetone inhibits ATPase activity, whereas ether appears to activate it. In contrast to the action of these solvents, aqueous heptane treatment does not cause inhibition of either calcium uptake or ATPase activity. The chief effect of heptane treatment of vesicles is thought to be the removal of cholesterol and other neutral lipids. From this evidence, it appears that these components are not very important in the functioning of this system.

An alternative method that has been used in studying the role of membrane lipids involves replacing endogenous lipids with defined exogenous lipids. Such substitution experiments have involved dioleoyl lecithin, dimyristoyl lecithin, dipalmitoyl lecithin [24-26], unsaturated fatty acids [73], and oleate and lysolecithin [74]. While all these agents have been shown to cause a reactivation of ATPase activity, only dioleoyl lecithin causes calcium pump activity to be restored. Thus the variety of phospholipids found in the FSR vesicles (and the purified ATPase) is not required for ATP hydrolysis or calcium transport. Unsaturated fatty acids with a chain length C_{16} to C_{18}, containing double bonds in the middle of the chain, were found to be most effective in restoring calcium-sensitive ATPase activity to delipated FSR membranes. Optimal activity was achieved with 70-106 molecules of fatty acid per 100,000-dalton ATPase protein unit. All the reconstituted preparations howed little activity at basic pH values [73].

Other studies [74] have indicated that while lipids are apparently not needed for ATP binding, they are significant in phosphoprotein formation. This is supported by data showing that phosphoprotein formation is stimulated if oleate is added to lipid-depleted vesicles and reduced if lysolecithin is added instead of oleate.

Data on the rates of lateral diffusion of phosphatidylcholine and phosphatidylethanolamine in FSR vesicles have been obtained by Devaux and McConnell [75]. Both lipids show a diffusion constant of about 7×10^{-8} cm^2/sec at 40 °C. This is close to what is seen in lecithin bilayers, and indicates that interaction of the bulk of the lipid molecules with the membrane ATPase protein molecules does not greatly affect their rates of lateral diffusion.

Membrane lipids have been shown to be prominent in both active calcium binding and passive calcium binding [76]. Calcium actively bound in the presence of ATP is released from FSR vesicles on treatment with either phospholipase A or phospholipase C. Such treatment also has the effect of increasing the passive cation-binding capacity of the membrane. This increase depends, however, on the presence of the degradation products of the phospholipids, since their removal decreases the binding capacity to about 50% of the initial value. It is thus apparent that membrane phospholipids account for a large fraction of the cation-binding capacity of FSR vesicles. Following extraction with 90% acetone, the cation-binding capacity of the membrane is reduced to 40% of its initial value but the apparently passive calcium-binding affinity is not affected by the lipid removal.

An interesting alteration in the normal pattern of lipid distribution has been observed in an investigation comparing the lipid compositions of normal and dystrophic FSR vesicles [77]. Dystrophic vesicles contain a significantly higher amount of cholesterol and a lower amount of lecithin, expressed per unit of membrane protein, than normal vesicles do (Table 5). This difference may be related to a structural alteration in FSR membranes, as reported by Baskin and Hanna [55].

Recent studies that resulted in the reconstitution of calcium transport from partially solubilized components [78] showed a requirement for added phosphatidylethanolamine; added phosphatidylcholine alone did not allow reconstitution of transport. The "purified" Ca^{2+}-Mg^{2+} ATPase did contain

TABLE 5

Lipid Composition of Normal and Dystrophic FSR

	Normal (mg lipid/100 mg protein)	Dystrophic (mg lipid/100 mg protein)
Phosphatidylcholine	21.7	13.8
Phosphatidylethanolamine	8.7	9.7
Phosphatidylserine	1.7	3.7
Sphingomyelin	3.8	8.9
Cardiolipin	2.6	2.3
Total phospholipid	40.8	40.7
Cholesterol	6.1	16.4
Triglycerides	6.1	12.6
Total neutral lipid	12.2	29.0
Total lipid	53.0	69.7

Source: Data of Hsu and Kaldor [77].

about 25% of the original lipids. This same preparation, containing a large amount of added phospholipid, was not permeable to oxalate, ATP, or Pi. The initial FSR vesicles were permeable to all these components.

Lipid removal studies using the detergent cholate and performed on a preparation of purified ATPase indicate that the detergent cannot easily remove the last 15 lipid molecules around each molecule of the enzyme [24-26]. For enzymatic activity to be maintained, a lipid-protein molar ratio of over 30 is required. This ratio would probably allow a single bilayer shell of lipids to surround the protein if it is assumed to have a diameter in the membrane of about 40 Å. This estimate, however, requires approximately 55% of the protein to extend outward from the membrane surface, a requirement that appears quite severe. An alternative explanation would be to postulate a lipid requirement for only certain folded regions of the polypeptide chain. Distortion of the chain and loss of activity would result from removal of these "critical" lipid molecules.

VI. THE BINDING OF CALCIUM

The interaction of calcium with the Ca^{2+}-Mg^{2+} ATPase protein has been shown to involve ATP and Mg^{2+} [79, 80]. Ebashi originally postulated that calcium transport resulted from the binding of calcium to receptor sites made accessible to calcium by ATP [81]. ATP-mediated binding of calcium to FSR membranes was considered an explanation for the rapid initial rate of calcium uptake measured by a rapid mixing technique [82].

Fragmented sarcoplasmic reticulum membranes show a cation-binding capacity of about 350 $\mu eq/g$ of protein at neutral pH [83]. The same binding sites bind Ca^{2+}, Mg^{2+}, K^+, and H^+ ions. Selective binding of calcium induced by ATP would release an equivalent amount of other cations. At pH values below 6.2, numerous binding sites are associated with H^+, and ATP induces exchange of Ca^{2+} for H^+. Above 6.2, the binding sites exist in the form of Mg^{2+} and K^+; Ca^{2+} is bound in exchange for these ions. To obtain the same amount of exchange of calcium for other cations bound in the absence of ATP requires a concentration of calcium higher by a thousandfold than is needed in the presence of ATP. Adenosine triphosphate (10^{-5} to 10^{-4} M) is required for the exchange of the "intrinsic" bound calcium and the "actively" bound calcium with calcium added to the medium [84]. The selective interaction of calcium with FSR membranes could arise either from a selectivity of binding sites to calcium induced by ATP or from the ATP-dependent active transport of calcium followed by attachment to intravesicular binding sites [84, 85].

Total cation-binding capacity has also been estimated on the basis of measurements of electrophoretic mobility of FSR membranes [86]. The resulting value, 70 $\mu eq/g$, is an estimate of the surface cation-binding capacity only. Internal binding sites would not be detected by this technique even if the membrane were completely permeable to all cations.

Calcium-binding sites in FSR membranes have been found to be associated both with the Ca^{2+}-Mg^{2+} ATPase protein and with calsequestrin [87-89]. Earlier studies had shown the presence of both low-affinity and high-affinity calcium binding sites [90, 91]. One category of sites (nonspecific) bound Ca^{2+} with a dissociation constant of 0.32 mM in the absence of KCl or $MgCl_2$ but not in their presence. With KCl and $MgCl_2$ present, a high-affinity binding site (dissociation constant = 1.2 μM) containing 10-20 nmole of Ca^{2+} per mg protein and a low-affinity site (dissociation constant = 40 μM) containing 90 nmole of Ca^{2+} per mg protein were found. Using a purified ATPase preparation, Ikemoto [92] has identified three types of binding sites, all of which, he assumes, are on the ATPase protein itself. In the absence of ATP, there is approximately one of each type of binding site per 10^5-dalton protein molecule. The estimated binding constants are 4×10^6 M^{-1} (alpha site), 4×10^4 M^{-1} (beta site), and 1×10^3 M^{-1} (gamma site). Adding 1.5 mM ATP increases the affinity of all sites and reduces the apparent capacity of the alpha and beta sites. Calcium binding at the alpha site activates ATP hydrolysis, whereas binding to the gamma site inhibits it. The beta site does not appear to be involved in ATP hydrolysis.

Meissner [93], using partially purified calcium pump protein (ATPase), studied ATP and calcium binding. He determined that the purified ATPase bound approximately 14 nmole of Ca^{2+} per mg protein (dissociation constant $\simeq$ 2 μM). Following from a presumed initial ATP and calcium-binding step, he concluded that the ATPase protein contains one specific high-affinity ATP-binding sites and two specific high-affinity calcium-binding sites per (protein) active site. An increase in the ATP and Ca^{2+} binding affinities was found with increasing pH. An Mg^{2+} binding site comparable in affinity with the ATP- and calcium-binding sites was missing from the unphosphorylated ATPase.

Chaotropic anions, which have long been known to inhibit calcium binding [8], have recently been shown to inhibit ATP binding also [94]. It was suggested that they interfere at the ATP-binding site by binding to a strategic region of the ATPase molecule.

In considering the role of calcium binding to the Ca^{2+}-Mg^{2+} ATPase protein, one must remember that intact SR (at least in the case of rabbit muscle preparations) has been shown to contain a calcium-sequestering protein (calsequestrin) and a high-affinity calcium-binding protein [88, 89]. Calsequestrin, an acidic protein with an approximate molecular weight of 46,000 daltons, binds up to 970 nmole of Ca^{2+} per mg protein with a dissociation constant of about 50 to 70 μM in the absence of KCl and 700 to 800 μM in the presence of KCl. The "high-affinity calcium-binding protein" is a soluble, acidic molecule with a molecular weight of approximately 55,000 daltons. It binds one mole of calcium per mole of protein with a dissociation constant of about 3 μM.

Calcium binding and release in FSR vesicles has been shown to be pH-dependent [86, 95]. Increasing the pH in a solution containing calcium-"loaded" vesicles resulted in the release of 80–90 nmole of calcium for a change of about 1.4 pH units. A decrease in pH of approximately 1.1 units resulted in a rebinding of 25–30 nmole of calcium per mg protein. Comparable studies have not as yet been performed on purified Ca^{2+}-Mg^{2+} ATPase protein and so it is not possible to determine the actual calcium sites that were sensitive to pH change in these experiments.

VII. PHOSPHOENZYME FORMATION AND THE HYDROLYSIS OF ATP

The hydrolysis of ATP by the Ca^{2+}-Mg^{2+} ATPase requires the presence of both Ca^{2+} and Mg^{2+} [5]. This hydrolysis, under suitable conditions, is accompanied by the transport of calcium and represents the energy source for this transport. The moles of calcium transported per mole of ATP hydrolyzed (Ca/ATP ratio) appeared to be quite variable, but with present techniques the ratio Ca to ATP is now generally considered 2:1 [14, 85, 96]. The rate of ATP hydrolysis is influenced by the free Ca^{2+} concentration in the medium [97–99]. Since both ATP hydrolysis and calcium transport activity show approximately the same dependence on external free calcium concentration [6, 7, 100], the Ca/ATP ratio is largely independent of free calcium concentration.

Fragmented sarcoplasmic reticulum vesicles have long been known to catalyze a phosphate exchange reaction between ATP and ADP [101–103]. This reaction shows a dependence on free calcium concentration similar to that shown by calcium transport activity and ATP hydrolysis. Half-maximal

activation of all three processes is reached at about 10^{-7} M free calcium [7].
ATPase activity, ATP-ADP exchange, and calcium transport are linked
through the formation of a phosphoprotein intermediate discovered by Yamamoto and Tonomura [104] and by Makinose [105]. The phosphoprotein intermediate was demonstrated following incubation of FSR vesicles with ^{32}P-ATP.
Protein-bound ^{32}P activity was found in the membrane. The phosphoprotein
intermediate was stable at acid pH and was rapidly hydrolyzed at alkaline pH
or in the presence of hydroxylamine [16, 104, 105]. This behavior indicated
an acylphosphate compound.

A new method for identifying and characterizing an acyl-phosphate linkage was developed by Degani and Boyer [106]. [^{3}H] Borohydride reduction of
the phosphorylated Ca^{2+}-Mg^{2+} ATPase followed by analysis of the acid
hydrolysate of the reduced enzyme showed the formation of labeled homo-
serine. This demonstrated that the FSR ATPase phosphoryl group was
attached to the β-carboxyl group of an aspartyl residue at the active site.

The steady-state level of the intermediate in the presence of 5 mM
$MgCl_2$ is less than 0.1 μmole per gram of protein. Adding 0.01 to 1.0 μmole
of calcium causes a rapid increase in the steady-state concentration of the
intermediate 1-4 μmole per gram of protein. (Since these values were calculated on the basis of total vesicle protein, the true steady-state levels per
mole of Ca^{2+}-Mg^{2+} ATPase protein would be higher.)

A reaction sequence showing a possible scheme for the interaction of
phosphoenzyme production, ATP hydrolysis, and calcium transport is shown
in Figure 9. The Ca^{2+}-Mg^{2+} ATPase protein (E) binds with 2 Ca^{2+} and
$MgATP^{2-}$ to form an $E_{Ca^{2+}-MgATP^{2-}}$ complex, which is considered a direct
precursor of the phosphorylated intermediate [93]. Binding of Ca^{2+} and
$MgATP^{2-}$ appears to follow a random sequence [93, 107]. Furthermore,
there is a linear relation between the reciprocals of the square of the free
calcium concentration and the maximum initial rate of phosphoenzyme formation, indicating according to Kanazawa et al. [107], a requirement for
two Ca^{2+} for phosphoenzyme formation.

Mg^{2+}-ATP bound to a protein-calcium complex accounts for one of the
roles of Mg^{2+} in the phosphorylation reaction. It may also be required for
phosphorylation and is believed to have a role in activating the breakdown
of the phosphoenzyme intermediate [93, 105, 107, 108]. Yamamoto [109]
concluded that the affinity of the ATPase protein for Ca^{2+} and Mg^{2+} changes
on phosphorylation, so that ATP hydrolysis goes to completion only following
an Mg^{2+}-dependent dephosphorylation. This result, in conjunction with studies
on an Mg^{2+}-dependent Pi $\leftrightarrows$ HOH exchange [101], indicates that Mg^{2+} is the
counterion for calcium transport. Calcium is thus transported in on one form
of the phosphorylated protein and Mg^{2+} is transported out on another. As a
result of this process, Mg^{2+}, ADP, and Pi would be released on the membrane exterior and calcium on the interior [20].

Meissner [93], following consideration of the evidence, has concluded
that the ATP binding site is present at the phosphorylation site, since (1) the

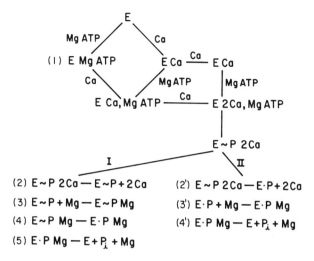

(2) E~P 2Ca — E~P+2Ca   (2') E~P 2Ca — E·P+2Ca

(3) E~P+Mg — E~P Mg   (3') E·P+Mg — E·P Mg

(4) E~P Mg — E·P Mg   (4') E·P Mg — E+P_i+Mg

(5) E·P Mg — E+P_i+Mg

FIG. 9 Reaction sequence showing a possible scheme for the interaction of phosphoenzyme production, ATP hydrolysis, and calcium transport. The Ca^{2+}-Mg^{2+} ATPase protein (E) binds with 2 Ca^{2+} and $MgATP^{2-}$ to form an $E_{Ca^{2+}-MgATP^{2-}}$ complex, which is considered to be a direct precursor of the phosphorylated intermediate. Binding of Ca^{2+} and $MgATP^{2-}$ appears to follow a random sequence. Following the formation of E ~ P2Ca, two alternative reaction sequences are indicated. Sequence I shows the transition E ~ P → E · P, where E · P represents a bound phosphate state, occurring during an Mg^{2+} transport step, while Sequence II shows this transition occurring following the release of calcium. Present evidence does not preferentially support either of these sequences.

$$E+S \underset{(1)}{\rightleftharpoons} ES \underset{(2)}{\rightleftharpoons} E{\sim}P \underset{(3)}{\rightleftharpoons} E{\cdot}P \underset{(4)}{\rightleftharpoons} E+P_i$$

$K_1 = 10^7\ m^{-1}s^{-1}$ $K_{-1} = 200\ s^{-1}$

$K_2 = 150\ s^{-1}$ $K_{-2} = 50\ s^{-1}$

$^*K_3 = 50\ s^{-1}$ $^*K_{-3} = 45\ s^{-1}$

$^*K\ =\ 10\ s^{-1}$

---

*For ATP > 10μM

FIG. 10 Kinetic scheme proposed by Froehlich and Taylor [112] to account for kinetics of formation of E · P over a restricted concentration range. Since a single set of rate constants can account for the kinetic data, only one class of site need be present to account for the steps leading to the E ~ P state.

number of ATP binding sites appears to be equal to the number of phosphoryl-ation sites, (2) phosphoenzyme formation blocks ATP binding, (3) phospho-enzyme formation and ATP binding are both optimal in the presence of Mg^{2+}, (4) inhibiting ATP binding results in a loss of phosphoenzyme formation, and (5) ATP binding is specific.

While phosphoenzyme formation requires calcium, adding Na^+ or K^+ at low ATP concentrations inhibits this formation, most likely by competing with calcium for its binding site [111]. The degree of inhibition varies with ATP concentration and temperature.

Froehlich and Taylor [112], using a rapid quenching method, have analyzed the transient-state behavior of FSR ATP hydrolysis. The simplest mechanism that could explain their kinetic data (Fig. 10) required two phosphate-containing intermediate states, a phosphorylated protein E ~ P, and a bound phosphate state E · P. It was apparent, however, that this scheme would not account for the kinetics of formation of EP over the entire concentration range. Estimated rate constants are given in Figure 10.

VIII. ATPase ACTIVITY

Absolute values of ATPase activity in different investigations have tended to vary widely. In some cases, ATPase activity was measured over many minutes when in fact ATP or some other component clearly became limiting after one or two minutes. Some estimates of purity were expressed as the percentage increase in ATPase activity in the purified preparation as con-trasted with the FSR preparation. This measure would, of course, depend on the purity of the initial preparation. Table 6 shows the values obtained by

TABLE 6

ATPase Activity of FSR and Purified Ca^{2+}-Mg^{2+} ATPase Preparations (μmoles/min-mg)

	FSR	ATPase	"Purification"
Martonosi [22]	3.5–5.0[a]	4.0[a]	
MacLennan [19]	10[a]	30[a]	3X
Meissner et al. [15]	1.0	5.5	5X
Deamer [28]	1.2–2.0	2.1	2X
Warren et al. [25]	2.6[a]	8.3[a]	3X
Baskin (Lobster FSR and ATPase purified by method of MacLennan [19]	2.36	4.68	2X

[a]Measured at 37 °C; other measurements at 23–26 °C.

numerous investigators for the ATPase activity of both the initial and the purified preparations. The highest value for the purified ATPase at 37 °C was reported by MacLennan [19] to be approximately 30 μmoles per min-mg. Meissner et al. [15] and Baskin (see Table 6) have obtained values around 5 μmoles per min-mg at 23 °C.

Half-maximal activation occurs between 0.2 and 1.0 μM calcium concentration with inhibition of the ATPase activity appearing at $[Ca^{2+}]$ of 0.1 to 1 mM [113-115]. The Ca^{2+}-Mg^{2+} ATPase has an apparent Km of 4×10^{-4} M; however, in the presence of an ATP regenerating system, it displays a greater affinity for ATP with an apparent Km between 0.7×10^{-6} M and 1×10^{-5} M.

As Meissner et al. [15] have pointed out, however, calcium transport and ATPase activity are partly dependent on the intactness of the membrane. Since this most likely varies from preparation to preparation, the reason for the discrepancies in measured values of ATPase activity become apparent. The best indicator of the purity of an ATPase preparation appears to be the measurement of phosphoenzyme content. If we assume a molecular weight of approximately 106,000 daltons, and the presence of one phosphorylation site per molecule, a pure preparation would show a phosphoenzyme content of 10 nmole per mg protein. Meissner et al. [15] have obtained preparations estimated to be 90% pure (9 nmole PE per mg protein) by treatment of a purified FSR preparation with bile acids in the presence of salt.

Evidence for the presence of one active site per ATPase molecule was provided by a study of Lineweaver-Burk plots of activated ATPase over a wide range of substrate concentrations [116]. The results indicated that the ATPase has one active site that used MgATP as its substrate and can be modified by free Mg^{2+}.

Allosteric inhibition of both calcium transport and ATPase activity by alkali ions (Li, K, Na) has been observed [117]. The pattern of the inhibition was a function of ATP concentration and the results were interpreted as indicating that the binding of ATP to the Ca^{2+} carrier system promotes conformational changes that result in a modification of its affinity for Ca^{2+}.

IX. CALCIUM TRANSPORT

The Ca^{2+}-Mg^{2+} ATPase protein is able to maintain the free Ca^{2+} concentration of the muscle sarcoplasm at a level of less than 10^{-7} M. As a result of the calcium transport process, the major portion of muscle calcium is stored within the sarcoplasmic reticulum. Calcium is present inside the sarcoplasmic reticulum at a concentration approximately 10^3 times greater than on the outside. Calcium transport occurs both in the presence of precipitating agents such as oxalate and in their absence.

Many experiments designed to measure uptake kinetics and the calcium uptake capacity of FSR vesicles have given ambiguous results. Three main sources of error exist. First, care must be taken to exclude the possibility of calcium phosphate precipitation, especially in measurements extending over many minutes. Secondly, it is difficult to avoid partial aggregation of the FSR vesicles, and aggregation may affect both calcium capacity and the kinetics of calcium uptake because of the effective reduction of membrane surface area. Finally, measurements of the velocity of calcium uptake in the absence of a precipitating agent do not differentiate between binding of calcium and actual transport. The experiments of Ohnishi and Ebashi [82] and of Ebashi and Ebashi [118] gave velocities of calcium uptake as high as 60 μmole per min–mg and probably include a combination of binding and transport.

The maximum rate of calcium uptake in the absence of a precipitating agent varies from preparation to preparation. Values range from 0.8 to 3.0 μmole per min–mg [6, 85, 98].

The calcium capacity in the absence of oxalate has been measured by various investigators and values between 0.1 and 0.5 μmole per mg have been reported [6, 119]. The level of steady-state filling depends on the pCa of the medium and shows maximum values between pCa = 6 and pCa = 7 [119].

In the presence of oxalate, rates of calcium uptake of about 1 to 4 μmole per mg–min (25 °C) have been obtained [7, 48, 85, 98]. The transport system exhibits saturation behavior between pCa = 8 and 6. Half-maximal activation occurs at a pCa of approximately 7. Measurement of calcium uptake and splitting of ATP over a broad range of ATP concentrations indicated that the hydrolysis of one mole resulted in the uptake of two moles of Ca^{2+}. This was shown to hold true even during early stages of calcium uptake in the absence of oxalate [120]. This ratio is independent of the calcium ion concentration gradient and indicates the interdependence of calcium transport and ATP hydrolysis. The calcium uptake capacity (in the presence of oxalate) was reported to be in excess of 8 μmole per mg protein [6], and we have measured capacities exceeding 17 μmole per mg in lobster muscle FSR [45].

The calcium uptake process is, interestingly, not specific for ATP. Other nucleotide triphosphates can substitute for ATP [6, 98, 121, 122]— ITP, GTP, CTP, and UTP all support calcium transport although at lower rates than ATP. Acetyl-phosphate and p-nitrophenyl phosphate can also be used as substrates for calcium transport [123, 124].

Sumida and Tonomura [125] investigated the time course of calcium uptake and compared it with the time course of formation and the time course of decomposition of the phosphorylated intermediate. They concluded that the time course of calcium uptake consisted of two phases: a rapid initial phase coupled with the formation of the phosphorylated intermediate, and a slow steady phase coupled with decomposition of the phosphorylated intermediate. Calcium ions taken up during the initial phase were released when EGTA was added to the medium. Those taken up during the steady state were insensitive to EGTA addition.

A recent study by Shamoo and MacLennan [126] has indicated that the Ca^{2+}-Mg^{2+} ATPase contains a calcium-dependent ionophore. Their evidence suggested that a small peptide with a high specificity for calcium is an integral part of the ATPase protein. The specific nature of the transport mediator (carrier or channel) was not indicated by this study.

X. REVERSIBLE MECHANISM FOR CALCIUM TRANSPORT

A hypothetical model for calcium transport is presented in Figure 11. As indicated earlier, Ca^{2+} and MgATP bind randomly to the enzyme in the ratio of 1 mole of ATP to 1 mole protein and 2 moles of Ca^{2+} to 1 mole protein. This probably occurs at the outer membrane surface and results in the

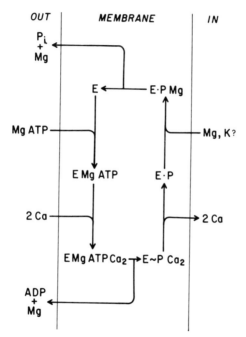

FIG. 11 A hypothetical model for calcium transport. Ca^{2+} and MgATP bind randomly to the Ca^{2+}-Mg^{2+} ATPase protein (E) in the ratio of 1 mole ATP to 1 mole protein and 2 moles Ca^{2+} to 1 mole protein. This occurs at the outer membrane surface and results in the release of Mg^{2+} and ADP. Translocation of the complex occurs and calcium is released to the interior. Following this release, E ~ P → E · P (a bound phosphate state). The complex next binds Mg^{2+} and translocates it to the exterior, where it and Pi are released.

release of Mg^{2+} and ADP. Translocation of the complex occurs and calcium
is released to the interior. Following this release of calcium, E ~ P is converted to E · P. (While evidence for this is lacking at present, Froehlich and
Taylor [112] have indicated that it should be forthcoming.) As a result of this
transition, the complex has an increased affinity for Mg^{2+}, which binds to it
and is translocated to the exterior, where it and Pi are released. Since the
process would be reversible, however, Kanazawa and Boyer [110] consider
that an oxygen exchange (Pi $\rightleftarrows$ HOH) may occur, that is, the formation of an
enzyme · Pi complex in the presence of Mg^{2+} and the formation of a covalent
enzyme–phosphate bond with elimination of water. (FSR vesicles were found
to catalyze a rapid Pi $\rightleftarrows$ HOH exchange in the presence of Mg^{2+} and in the
absence of ATP and Ca^{2+}. The reaction required the integrity of the membrane, since it was inhibited by the addition of Triton X-100. The possibility
exists, however, that this inhibition was due to the release of internal calcium
by the detergent, although the presence of EGTA would appear to make this
unlikely.)

XI. RECONSTITUION OF TRANSPORT SYSTEM

Attempts to reconstitute the calcium transport system were made following
the initial solubilization of the ATPase. Martonosi [22] was able to obtain
some calcium transport activity in "regenerated microsomes" following an
initial extraction with deoxycholate and subsequent removal of the detergent.
He subsequently pointed out, however [9], that the partial restoration of
calcium transport may represent reassociation of previously undisrupted
membrane fragments and not a reassembly of functionally competent membranes from molecularly dispersed constituents. The extremely active
ATPase obtained by MacLennan [19] following use of deoxycholate and salt
fractionation showed only a low rate of calcium binding. The lysolecithin-
ATPase complex isolated by Deamer [28] did not show any evidence of
calcium transport.

The actual expression of calcium transport, however, requires not only
an active Ca^{2+}–Mg^{2+} ATPase protein but also that the integrity of the membrane be maintained. Another factor is the possible requirement of one or
more calcium–binding proteins. The highly active purified ATPase obtained
by Warren et al. [26] cannot accumulate calcium. Following a sedimentation-
substitution technique and the replacement of 99% of the ATPase lipid with
dioleoyl lecithin, restoration of the calcium transport can be achieved by
adding excess lipids in the presence of cholate and subsequently removing the
cholate by dialysis. This procedure results in a level of calcium-transport
activity comparable with the initial FSR preparation. This experiment also
shows quite clearly that the Ca^{2+}–Mg^{2+} ATPase protein molecule contains
both the site of ATP hydrolysis and the calcium carrier.

Meissner and Fleischer [127] solubilized FSR vesicles using deoxycholate. Following removal of the detergent by dialysis, energized calcium transport could be observed, though at a reduced level. These investigators found that two other proteins with a molecular weight in the range of 55,000 daltons (calcium-binding and M$_{55}$ proteins) were only partially rebound, perhaps explaining the lower calcium transport activity.

Reconstitution of a calcium pump using the Ca^{2+}-Mg^{2+} ATPase of MacLennan has been achieved in two somewhat different ways. The first involves combining the ATPase with soybean phospholipids in the presence of cholate [128]. Following dialysis of the solution against a phosphate buffer, a preparation with low calcium uptake activity resulted. The second method involves combining the ATPase with a preparation of purified phospholipids and sonication of the mixture for several minutes. This "detergent-free" method resulted in the reconstitution of vesicles with a substantial calcium transport ability [129]. In a recent study, Knowles and Racker [78] obtained a reconstituted preparation using the Ca^{2+}-Mg^{2+} ATPase and various phospholipids (their composition could be varied). This preparation not only showed a high level of calcium transport activity but also allowed the demonstration of pump reversal and the production of ATP. The reconstituted vesicles in this preparation were impermeable to oxalate, ATP and Pi, allowing a demonstration of calcium transport without the entry of the terminal phosphate of ATP into the interior of the vesicle.

XII. ATP SYNTHESIS BY THE Ca^{2+}-Mg^{2+} ATPase PROTEIN

It is important in considering possible mechanisms of calcium transport [96] to determine whether the transport system is reversible or not. The chemiosmotic coupling of ion transport to ATP hydrolysis as discussed by Mitchell [130] involves a reversible process. Evidence indicating a reversal of ATP hydrolysis in FSR has been presented by Makinose and Hasselbach [131] and by Panet and Selinger [132]. Earlier work by Kanazawa et al. [107] had shown that ATP could be formed from ADP and the phosphorylated intermediate. Makinose and Hasselbach and Panet and Selinger [131, 132] demonstrated the coupling between calcium translocation and the phosphoryl transfer reaction. Potential energy, they concluded, in the form of an osmotically inert calcium phosphate precipitate can serve as the driving force for ATP synthesis. Furthermore, it can do this with a high degree of efficiency. one molecule of ATP being synthesized per two Ca^{2+} translocated. Deamer and Baskin [96], by altering the permeability of FSR membranes, showed the absence of an obligatory coupling between calcium transport and ionic gradients, thus ruling out a Mitchell type of chemiosmotically linked mechanism. Their evidence was consistent with a transport mechanism in which inward transport is tightly coupled to phosphorylation of a transport enzyme by ATP. In the presence of a calcium gradient, FSR membranes are able to catalyze synthesis of ATP, apparently by a reversal of the inward transport reactions.

Support for this hypothesis was presented by the work of Makinose [133] and of Yamada et al. [134], which showed the formation of a phosphoenzyme (PE) intermediate during the calcium-driven synthesis of ATP. This PE intermediate was indistinguishable from that formed during active calcium accumulation. The time course of PE formation when FSR vesicles are preloaded with Ca^{2+} was determined by Yamada and Tonomura [135].

The formation of a high-energy PE in the absence of nucleoside triphosphate or a concentration gradient has been shown by Masuda and De Meis [136]. This reaction was strongly inhibited by Ca^{2+} and to a lesser extent by Na^+ and K^+. ATP and ADP competed with orthophosphate for the membrane phosphorylating sites. It was suggested that nucleoside triphosphates and orthophosphate interact with the same site on the membrane and that the binding of calcium determines which of them will phosphorylate the membrane. Further studies [137] showed that FSR membranes could be phosphorylated by orthophosphate through two different reactions. One of these reactions was strongly inhibited by Ca^{2+} and was not modified when ATP, ITP, or GTP was added to the assay medium. The other reaction is observed in the presence of Ca^{2+} and requires ITP, GTP, or ATP as a cofactor. FSR vesicles have also been shown to catalyze a calcium-dependent exchange reaction between orthophosphate and the α-phosphate of ATP. This exchange occurs both in the presence and in the absence of a transmembrane calcium gradient [138].

ATP formation from ADP and Pi without, apparently, the formation of an ion gradient across the membrane has been shown by Knowles and Racker [139]; they used vesicles formed from the purified Ca^{2+}-Mg^{2+} ATPase. The formation of a PE by these vesicles in the presence of Pi and Mg^{2+} was shown initially. When ADP and Ca^{2+} were added, most of the phosphate bound to the enzyme was transferred to form ATP. The ATP that was formed was not tightly bound to the enzyme but was free in solution. It was suggested that the energy for ATP formation was derived from the interaction of Ca^{2+} with the protein.

While it is known that the vesicles formed from the purified Ca^{2+}-Mg^{2+} ATPase do not transport calcium, the reason for this is not clear. It may be because the vesicles are "leaky" [78], or it may be due to the altered position of the ATPase protein in the membrane, as postulated earlier. While the existence of an ion gradient across the membrane appears to be ruled out, the absolute requirement for Mg^{2+} and its part in this reaction are not clear. The hypothesis is that the energy for ATP formation is derived from the interaction of Ca^{2+} with the protein [139], and it will undoubtedly receive further study. It appears to be consistent with the hypothesis of Boyer et al. [140], which considers the existence of "preformed" ATP at a catalytic site. Release of this ATP could involve an energy-requiring conformational change.

XIII. SUMMARY

The Ca^{2+}-Mg^{2+} ATPase protein can be obtained with a complement of lipid by either the MacLennan technique [19] or by the method of Warren et al. [24-26]. A single ATPase protein molecule probably contains approximately 30 tightly bound lipid molecules whose removal results in the denaturation of the protein. The protein-plus-lipid complex may exist in the membrane as a spheroid or ellipsoid structure. The evidence suggests that it is asymmetrically located in the membrane, most likely centered nearer the outer edge of the bilayer. A portion of the molecule containing the active site lies at the membrane surface or extends beyond it. While the ATPase is an "intrinsic" membrane protein, it has an amphipathic character. Its hydrophobic portion is within the phospholipid bilayer while its polar portion is at (or near) the membrane surface. This polar portion contains the site for the hydrolysis of ATP. In the membranes formed from the ATPase preparation alone, the protein appears to be symmetrically located within the bilayer and this altered position may affect the ability of the protein to transport calcium. What the proteolipid that is normally present in the ATPase preparation does is not known, but there is no evidence linking it or any of the extrinsic proteins to an obligatory role in transport. That over 30 percent of the amino acids composing the ATPase protein are strongly hydrophilic supports the idea that a considerable portion of the molecule extends past the membrane surface or lies along it.

While the 80-Å membrane particles seen following freeze-fracturing clearly represent the ATPase complex, the origin of the 40-Å surface particles observed following negative staining is less certain. They are most likely related to the presence of the ATPase protein and not to an extrinsic protein layer.

The effect of trypsin may be to cleave a portion of the ATPase molecule, resulting in the loss of the 40-Å particles, but it is also possible that trypsin alters the membrane structure in such a way that the 40-Å particles are not seen following negative staining. This idea is supported by the studies of Ikemoto et al. [43], who found that removal (or nonappearance) of the 40-Å particle did not affect calcium transport or ATPase activity.

The studies of Masuda and De Meis [136] and those of Knowles and Racker [139], both of which appear to show the formation of high-energy compounds in the absence of nucleoside triphosphates or an osmotic gradient, require further investigation. The precise nature of the energetic coupling that would allow such a formation is clearly of great interest to chemists and biologists.

ACKNOWLEDGMENTS

The support of NIH Grant No. HL-12978 for portions of this work is gratefully acknowledged.

REFERENCES

1. E. Veratti, Memorie Inst. Lomb Cl. Sci. e Nat., 19, 87 (1902).
2. B. B. Marsh, Biochim. Biophys. Acta, 9, 247-260 (1952).
3. J. R. Bendall, Nature, 107, 1058-1060 (1952).
4. S. Ebashi and F. Lipmann, J. Cell Biol., 14, 389-400 (1962).
5. W. Hasselbach and M. Makinose, Biochem. Z., 333, 518-528 (1961).
6. W. Hasselbach, Prog. Biophys. Biophys. Chem., 14, 167-222 (1964).
7. A. Weber, Current Topics in Bioenergetics, ed. P. R. Sanadi, Vol. 1. New York: Academic Press, 1966, p. 203-254.
8. S. Ebashi, M. Otsuka, and M. Endo, Excerpta Med. Int. Congr. Ser., 48, 899 (1962).
9. A. Martonosi, in Biomembranes, ed. L. A. Manson, Vol. 1. New York: Plenum, 1971, p. 191-256.
10. G. Inesi, Ann. Rev. Biophys. Bioeng., 1, 191-210 (1972).
11. H. Portzehl, Biochim. Biophys. Acta, 26, 373-377 (1957).
12. L. Lorand, J. Molnar, and C. Moos, in Conference of the Chemistry of Muscular Contraction Tokyo: Igaku-Shoin Ltd., 1957, p. 85.
13. A. Martonosi, Fed. Proc., 23, 913-921 (1964).
14. W. Hasselbach and M. Makinose, Biochem. Z., 339, 94-111 (1963).
15. G. Meissner, G. E. Conner, and S. Fleischer, Biochim. Biophys. Acta, 298, 246-269 (1973).
16. A. Martonosi, J. Biol. Chem., 244, 613-620 (1969).
17. A. Martonosi and R. A. Halpin, Arch. Biochem. Biophys., 144, 66-77 (1971).
18. D. H. MacLennan and P. T. S. Wong, Proc. Nat. Acad. Sci. U.S., 68, 1231-1235 (1971).
19. D. H. MacLennan, J. Biol. Chem., 245, 4508-4518 (1970).
20. D. H. MacLennan, Can. J. Biochem., 53, 251-261 (1975).
21. D. H. MacLennan, C. C. Yip, G. H. Iles, and P. Seaman, Cold Spring Harbor Sym., 37, 469-477 (1972).
22. A. Martonosi, J. Biol. Chem., 243, 71-81 (1968).
23. D. H. MacLennan, P. Seeman, G. H. Iles, and C. C. Yip, J. Biol. Chem., 246, 2702-2710 (1971).
24. G. B. Warren, N. J. M. Birdsall, A. G. Lee, and J. C. Metcalfe, in Membrane Proteins in Transport and Phosphorylation, ed. G. F. Azzone, M. E. Klingenberg, E. Quagliariello, and N. Siliprandi. Amsterdam: North-Holland Publishing Co., 1974, p. 1-12.
25. G. B. Warren, P. A. Toon, N. J. M. Birdsall, A. G. Lee, and J. C. Metcalfe, FEBS Letters, 41, 122-124 (1974).
26. G. B. Warren, P. A. Toon, N. J. M. Birdsall, A. G. Lee, and J. C. Metcalfe, Proc. Nat. Acad. Sci. U.S., 71, 622-626 (1974).
27. H. Walter and W. Hasselbach, Eur. J. Biochem., 36, 110-119 (1973).
28. D. W. Deamer, J. Biol. Chem., 248, 5477-5485 (1973).
29. B. P. Yu and E. J. Masoro, Biochem., 9, 2909-2917 (1970).

30. A. G. Purcell and A. Martonosi, Arch. Biochem. Biophys., 151, 558–564 (1972).
31. P. S. Stewart and D. H. MacLennan, J. Biol. Chem., 249, 985–993 (1974).
32. D. H. MacLennan, T. J. Ostwald, and P. S. Stewart, Ann. N.Y. Acad. Sci., 227, 527–536 (1974).
33. B. G. McFarland and G. Inesi, Arch. Biochim. Biophys., 145, 456–464 (1971).
34. D. W. Deamer and R. J. Baskin, J. Cell Biol., 42, 296–307 (1969).
35. J. D. Robertson, Ann. N.Y. Acad. Sci., 137, 421–440 (1966).
36. J. C. Selser, Y. Yeh, and R. J. Baskin, Biophysical J., 16, 337–356 (1976).
37. B. Agostini and W. Hasselbach, J. Submicr. Cytol., 3, 231–238 (1971).
38. H. E. Huxley, Proceedings of the Stockholm Conference on Electron Microscopy, 1956. Stockholm: Almquist and Wiksell, 1957, p. 260.
39. N. Ikemoto, F. A. Sreter, A. Nakamura, and J. Gergely, J. Ultrastruct. Res., 23, 216–232 (1968).
40. A. Martonosi, Biochim. Biophys. Acta, 150, 694–704 (1968).
41. P. Hardwicke and N. M. Green, Eur. J. Biochem., 42, 183–193 (1974).
42. W. Hasselbach and L. G. Elfvin, J. Ultrastruct. Res., 17, 598–622 (1967).
43. N. Ikemoto, F. A. Sreter, and J. Gergely, Arch. Biochem. Biophys., 147, 571–582 (1971).
44. R. J. Baskin and D. W. Deamer, J. Cell Biol., 43, 610–617 (1969).
45. R. J. Baskin, J. Cell Biol., 48, 49–60 (1971).
46. D. Branton, Proc. Nat. Acad. Sci. U.S., 55, 1048–1056 (1966).
47. N. E. Flower, J. Cell Sci., 12, 445–452 (1973).
48. R. J. Baskin, J. Ultrastruct. Res., 49, 348–371 (1974).
49. R. Boland and A. Martonosi, J. Biol. Chem., 249, 612–623 (1974).
50. W. J. Vail, D. Papahadjopoulos, and M. A. Moscarello, Biochem. Biophys. Acta, 345, 463–467 (1974).
51. D. A. Thorley-Lawson and N. M. Green, Eur. J. Biochem., 40, 403–413 (1973).
52. A. Migala, B. Agostini, and W. Hasselbach, Z. Naturforsch., 28, 178–182 (1973).
53. L. Packer, C. W. Mehard, G. Meissner, W. L. Zahler, and S. Fleischer, Biochim. Biophys. Acta, 363, 159–181 (1974).
54. R. J. Baskin, Lab. Invest., 23, 581–589 (1970).
55. R. J. Baskin and S. D. Hanna, The Physiologist, 18, 132 (1975).
56. C. R. Worthington and S. C. Liu, Arch. Biochem. Biophys., 157, 573–579 (1973).
57. S. C. Liu and C. R. Worthington, Arch. Biochem. Biophys., 163, 332–342 (1974).
58. Y. DuPont, S. C. Harrison, and W. Hasselbach, Nature, 244, 555–558 (1973).
59. Y. DuPont and W. Hasselbach, Nature New Biology, 246, 41–43 (1973).
60. L. Marai and A. Kuksis, Can. J. Biochem., 51, 1248–1261 (1973).

61. L. Marai and A. Kuksis, Can. J. Biochem., 51, 1365-1379 (1973).
62. A. Martonosi, Biochem. Biophys. Res. Commun., 13, 273-278 (1963).
63. G. Meissner and S. Fleischer, Biochim. Biophys. Acta, 241, 356-378 (1971).
64. G. B. Warren, P. A. Toon, N. J. M. Birdsall, A. G. Lee, and J. C. Metcalfe, Biochem. 13, no. 27, 5501-5507 (1974).
65. A. Martonosi, J. R. Donley, A. G. Purcell, and R. A. Halpin, Arch. Biochem. Biophys., 144, 529-540 (1971).
66. A. Martonosi, J. Donley, and R. A. Halpin, J. Biol. Chem., 243, 61-70 (1968).
67. J. B. Finean and A. Martonosi, Biochim. Biophys. Acta, 98, 547-553 (1965).
68. B. P. Yu, F. D. DeMartinis, and E. J. Masoro, J. Lipid Res., 9, 492-500 (1968).
69. W. Fiehn and W. Hasselbach, Eur. J. Biochem., 13, 510-518 (1970).
70. G. Inesi, J. J. Goodman, and S. Watanabe, J. Biol. Chem., 242, 4637-4643 (1967).
71. W. Fiehn and W. Hasselbach, Eur. J. Biochem., 9, 574-578 (1969).
72. W. Drabikowski, M. G. Sarzala, A. Wroniszewska, E. Lagwinska, and B. Drzewiecka, Biochim. Biophys. Acta, 274, 158-170 (1972).
73. R. The and W. Hasselbach, Eur. J. Biochem., 39, 63-68 (1973).
74. R. The and W. Hasselbach, Eur. J. Biochem., 28, 357-363 (1972).
75. P. Devaux and H. M. McConnell, Ann. New York Acad. Sci., 222, 487-498 (1973).
76. A. P. Carvalho, Eur. J. Biochem., 27, 491-502 (1972).
77. Q. S. Hsu and G. Kaldor, Proc. Soc. Exp. Biol. and Med., 138, 733-737 (1971).
78. A. F. Knowles and E. Racker, J. Biol. Chem., 250, 3538-3544 (1975).
79. S. Ebashi, J. Biochem. (Tokyo), 48, 150-151 (1960).
80. S. Ebashi, J. Biochem. (Tokyo), 50, 236-244 (1961).
81. S. Ebashi and M. Endo, in Biochemistry of Muscle Contraction, ed. J. Gergelt. Boston: Little, Brown, 1964, p. 199.
82. T. Ohnishi and S. Ebashi, J. Biochem. (Tokyo), 55, 599-603 (1964).
83. A. P. Carvalho and B. Leo, J. Gen. Physiol., 50, 1327-1352 (1967).
84. A. P. Carvalho, J. Gen. Physiol., 52, 622-642 (1968).
85. A. Weber, R. Herz, and I. Reiss, Biochem. Z., 354, 329-369 (1966).
86. R. J. Baskin, Bioenergetics, 3, 249-269 (1972).
87. N. Ikemoto, B. Nagy, G. M. Bhatnagar, and J. Gergely, J. Biol. Chem., 249, 2357-2365 (1974).
88. T. J. Ostwald and D. H. MacLennan, J. Biol. Chem., 249, 974-979 (1974).
89. T. J. Ostwald and D. H. MacLennan, J. Biol. Chem., 249, 5867-5871 (1974).
90. H. A. Bertrand, E. J. Masoro, T. Ohnishi and B. P. Yu, Biochemistry, 10, 3679-3685 (1971).

91. J. Chevallier and R. A. Butow, Biochemistry, 10, 2733-2737 (1971).
92. N. Ikemoto, J. Biol. Chem., 249, 649-651 (1974).
93. G. Meissner, Biochim. Biophys. Acta, 298, 906-926 (1973).
94. R. The and W. Hasselbach, Eur. J. Biochem., 53, 105-113 (1975).
95. Y. Nakamaru and A. Schwartz, J. Gen. Physiol., 59, 22-32 (1972).
96. D. W. Deamer and R. J. Baskin, Arch. Biochem. Biophys., 153, 47-54 (1972).
97. A. Martonosi and R. Feretos, Fed. Proc., 22, 35 (1963).
98. A. Martonosi and R. Feretos, J. Biol. Chem., 239, 648-658 (1964).
99. A. Martonosi and R. Feretos, J. Biol. Chem., 239, 659-668 (1964).
100. M. Makinose and W. Hasselbach, Biochem. Z., 343, 360-382 (1965).
101. G. Ulbrecht and M. Ulbrecht, Biochem. Biophys. Acta, 25, 100-109 (1957).
102. W. Hasselbach and M. Makinose, Biochem. Biophys. Res. Commun., 7, 132-136 (1962).
103. M. Makinose, Biochem. Z., 345, 80-86 (1966).
104. T. Yamamoto and Y. Tonomura, J. Biochem. (Tokyo), 64, 137-145 (1968).
105. M. Makinose, Eur. J. Biochem., 10, 74-82 (1969).
106. C. Degani and P. D. Boyer, J. Biol. Chem., 248, 8222-8226 (1973).
107. T. Kanazawa, S. Yamada, T. Yamamoto, and Y. Tonomura, J. Biochem. (Tokyo), 70, 95-123 (1971).
108. R. Panet, U. Pick, and Z. Selinger, J. Biol. Chem., 246, no. 23, 7349-7356 (1971).
109. T. Yamamoto, Muscle Proteins, Muscle Contraction, and Cation Transport, ed. Y. Tonomura. Baltimore: University Park Press, 1972, pp. 303-356.
110. T. Kanazawa and P. D. Boyer, J. Biol. Chem., 248, 3163-3172 (1973).
111. L. De Meis, Biochemistry, 11, 2460-2465 (1972).
112. J. P. Froehlich and E. W. Taylor, J. Biol. Chem., 250, 2013-2021 (1975).
113. A. Weber, J. Gen. Physiol., 57, 50-63 (1971).
114. T. Yamamoto and Y. Tonomura, J. Biochem. (Tokyo), 62, 558-575 (1967).
115. G. Inesi and J. Almendares, Arch. Biochem. Biophys., 126, 733-735 (1968).
116. D. J. Horgan, Arch. Biochem. Biophys., 162, 6-11 (1974).
117. L. De Meis, J. Biol. Chem., 246, 4764-4773 (1971).
118. S. Ebashi and F. Ebashi, J. Biochem. (Tokyo), 55, 604-613 (1964).
119. A. Weber, R. Herz, and I. Reiss, Proc. Roy. Soc. B, 160, 489-499 (1964).
120. S. Yamada, T. Yamamoto, and Y. Tonomura, J. Biochem. (Tokyo), 67, 789-794 (1970).
121. M. E. Carsten and W. F. H. M. Mommaerts, J. Gen. Physiol., 48, 183-197 (1964).

122. M. Makinose and R. The, Biochem. Z., 343, 383–393 (1965).
123. L. De Meis, Biochim. Biophys. Acta, 172, 343–344 (1969).
124. G. Inesi, Science (March, 1971), pp. 901–903 (1971).
125. M. Sumida and Y. Tonomura, J. Biochem. (Tokyo), 75, 283–297 (1974).
126. A. E. Shamoo and D. H. MacLennan, Proc. Nat. Acad. Sci. U.S.,
     71, 3522–3526 (1974).
127. G. Meissner and S. Fleischer, J. Biol. Chem., 249, 302–309 (1974).
128. E. Racker, J. Biol. Chem., 247, 8198–8200 (1972).
129. E. Racker and E. Eytan, Biochem. Biophys. Res. Commun., 55, 174–
     178 (1973).
130. P. Mitchell, Biol. Rev., 41, 445–502 (1966).
131. M. Makinose and W. Hasselbach, FEBS Letters, 12, 271–286 (1971).
132. R. Panet and Z. Selinger, Biochim. Biophys. Acta, 255, 34–42 (1972).
133. M. Makinose, FEBS Letters, 25, 113–115 (1972).
134. S. Yamada, M. Sumida, and Y. Tonomura, J. Biochem. (Tokyo), 72,
     1537–1548 (1972).
135. S. Yamada and Y. Tonomura, J. Biochem. (Tokyo), 74, 1091–1096 (1973).
136. H. Masuda and L. De Meis, Biochemistry, 12, 4581–4585 (1973).
137. L. De Meis and H. Masuda, Biochemistry, 13, 2057–2062 (1974).
138. L. De Meis and M. G. C. Carvalho, Biochemistry, 13, 5032–5038
     (1974).
139. A. F. Knowles and E. Racker, J. Biol. Chem., 250, 1949–1951 (1975).
140. P. D. Boyer, R. L. Cross, and W. Momsen, Proc. Nat. Acad. Sci.
     U.S., 70, 2837–2839 (1973).

Chapter 5

THE Na^+-K^+ ATPase

Ronald E. Barnett*

Department of Chemistry
University of Minnesota
Minneapolis, Minnesota

I. INTRODUCTION

Understanding the structure and function of mammalian-cell-membrane enzymes has been seriously hampered by the heterogeneity of the cell membrane and a lack of techniques for obtaining information about mechanism from a heterogeneous system. This is particularly true of attempts to define the features of lipid-protein interactions that may influence enzyme function.

One of the most thoroughly studied plasma membrane enzymes is the Na^+-K^+ ATPase. This enzyme has been shown to be responsible for actively transporting K^+ into the cell and Na^+ out [1-2]. The transport of ions is tightly coupled to ATP hydrolysis, as it is possible to synthesize ATP from ADP and phosphate using sodium and potassium ion concentration gradients [3-4]. In the red blood cell, two potassium ions are transported in and three sodium ions out per ATP hydrolyzed [5-6].

It is likely that the Na^+-K^+ ATPase protein extends entirely through the membrane. Adenosine triphosphate is hydrolyzed only if it is inside the cell

*Current affiliation: Department of Biochemistry and Nutrition, Virginia Polytechnic Institute and State University, Blacksburg, Virginia.

TABLE 1

Properties of the Purified $Na^+ - K^+$ ATPase from Various Sources

Detergent used	MW	Specific activity (μmoles ATP/hyd/mg protein/min)	Purity as esti-mated by authors	Glycopeptide (catalytic peptide)	Lipid bound	Ref.
Deoxycholate	$282,000^c$	13	90–100%	1.0	N.D.[a]	18
Lubrol	248,000	25	~100%	0.5	~50%[b]	19
Deoxycholate and lubrol	~100,000	120^d	~100%	0.0	67%–75%	21
Dodecyl sulfate	~249,000	37	~100%	0.5	50%	20

[a] Requires phosphatidyl serine for activity.
[b] Spin label studies suggest a lipid bilayer structure.
[c] Assuming two catalytic subunits/ATPase.
[d] Very labile.
[e] Assuming the glycopeptide is part of the ATPase.

[7], while the cardiac glycosides, such as ouabain, which are specific inhibitors of the Na^+-K^+ ATPase and of active transport, bind only on the outside [8]. Sodium ions must be on the inside of the cell and potassium ions on the outside to stimulate ATP hydrolysis [9]. The protein is large, with an estimated molecular weight of 250,000 [10].

There is some evidence that the Na^+-K^+ ATPase can interact with other proteins of the plasma membrane. The red blood cells of low potassium (LK) sheep possess antigenic sites (the L antigen) that influence V_{max} and K_m for K^+ [11]. When red blood cells of LK sheep are treated with anti-L antibody, both active transport and Na^+-K^+ ATPase activity are dramatically activated [12], the K_m for K^+ is decreased [13], and the rate of cardiac glycoside binding is increased [14]. Although binding of antibody is rapid, the effects on the ATPase and the transport system require 10-30 min to develop. Monovalent Fab fragments give no stimulation of transport activity, although pretreatment with monovalent Fab followed by antibody to Fab gives some stimulation of transport activity [11, 15]. These data suggest that after antibody binding, the antibody-receptor complex migrates laterally in the membrane [16], giving rise to multiple antibody-receptor complexes, which in turn result in activation of the transport system.

II. PURIFICATION AND PHYSICAL CHARACTERISTICS

Many of the recent advances in understanding the Na^+-K^+ ATPase are a result of the availability of highly purified preparations of the enzyme (Table 1). All procedures include a mild detergent treatment [17-21]. The specific activity of the purified enzyme is 13-120 μmole ATP hydrolyzed per mg protein per min. Most of the variability in specific activity is probably due to differences in turnover number [20] rather than differences in purity.

The best preparations of the Na^+-K^+ ATPase give two polypeptide bands on acrylamide gel-SDS electrophoresis [17-20]. Both polypeptides are homogeneous by end-group analysis, there being only one N-terminal amino acid for each band [18-19]. The larger polypeptide of molecular weight around 100,000 is the catalytic subunit. An aspartate residue of this polypeptide is phosphorylated by ATP to give an acyl phosphate [17-24]. The smaller polypeptide is a glycoprotein with molecular weight about 50,000 [17-20]. The role this polypeptide plays if any in ATPase activity remains to be decided. Cross-linking experiments using suberimidate indicate that the glycoprotein is in close proximity to the catalytic protein [18]. Yet the amount of glycoprotein found depends on the purification procedure used, and in one preparation it is apparently missing altogether [21].

The catalytic protein has 38%-39% hydrophobic amino acids for four different species, while the glycoprotein has 34%-35% hydrophobic residues for three species. The carbohydrate of the glycoprotein is quite species-dependent, both in amount and composition.

Two groups using quite different purification procedures report that there are two catalytic proteins per glycoprotein, giving an approximate molecular weight for the complex of 250,000 [19-20]. The molecular weight estimate obtained by X-ray inactivation of the ATPase is also 250,000 [10]. The maximum molecular weight based on ouabain binding is 282,000 for Jørgensen's preparation [20], which has a specific activity of 37 units per mg (one unit = one μmole ATP hydrolyzed per min).

III. MECHANISM

Although there is by no means a complete understanding of the mechanism of the Na^+-K^+ ATPase, many of the overall features are now understood. Several lines of evidence support a reaction scheme in which there is a Na^+-dependent phosphorylation to give $E_1 \sim P$, a conformational change to give $E_2 - P$, and K^+-dependent dephosphorylation of $E_2 - P$ [25]. The overall scheme is outlined in Eqs. (1)-(3). The phosphoenzyme exists in two states, which can be distinguished by their ability to transfer its phosphate to ADP [26-27]

$$E_1 + ATP \xrightleftharpoons{M^{2+}/Na^+} E_1 \sim P + ADP \tag{1}$$

$$E_1 \sim P \xrightleftharpoons{\hspace{1cm}} E_2 - P \tag{2}$$

$$E_2 - P \xrightleftharpoons{K^+} E + P_i \tag{3}$$

The E_1 form can transfer its phosphate but the E_2 form cannot. The two forms are both acyl phosphates with the phosphate on the same aspartate residue, and so $E_1 \sim P$ and $E_2 - P$ probably differ only in conformation [28]. Since $E_1 \sim P$ can transfer its phosphate to ADP, it is considered to be a "high-energy" phosphate. Since $E_2 - P$ can be formed from dephosphoenzyme and phosphate directly, it is a "low-energy" phosphate [29-31]. One of the most interesting but poorly understood aspects of the ATPase is the enormous effect of enzyme conformation on the thermodynamic stability of the phosphoenzyme. Since $E_1 \sim P$ can transfer its phosphate to ADP, the free energy of hydrolysis of $E_1 \sim P$ must be at least as negative as -7,000 to -8,000 cal/mole, the free energy of hydrolysis of ATP [32]. However, since $E_2 - P$ can be formed from enzyme plus phosphate, its free energy of hydrolysis must be near zero cal per mole. Thus, $E_2 - P$ must be "conformationally activated" and probably represents the point at which the chemical energy available from ATP hydrolysis is converted to mechanical energy for the transport of ions.

The formation of $E_1 \sim P$ requires a divalent metal ion. With Mg^{2+} or Mn^{2+}, $E_1 \sim P$ readily converts to $E_2 - P$ [26, 28]. The conversion can be blocked with SH reagents [33]. With Ca^{2+}, $E_1 \sim P$ can form but cannot be converted to $E_2 - P$ [27]. There appear to be several forms of $E_2 - P$: one that is rapidly dephosphorylated in the presence of K^+, one that is formed in the presence of ouabain, and one that is formed in the presence of Mg^{2+}

alone [25]. Each has its distinguishing characteristics, although their significance in the function of the ATPase is not well understood.

The step of Eq. (3) has not been the most thoroughly studied part of the ATPase mechanism. It can be further subdivided into 4 steps (Eqs. (4)-(7)), which can be isolated kinetically [25].

$$E_2 - P + K^+ \rightleftharpoons E_2 - P \cdot K^+ \tag{4}$$

$$E_2 - P \cdot K^+ \rightleftharpoons E_2 - K^+ + P_i \tag{5}$$

$$E_2 \cdot K^+ \rightleftharpoons E_2 + K^+ \tag{6}$$

$$E_2 \rightleftharpoons E_1 \tag{7}$$

With the availability of relatively pure ATPase preparations, it has been possible to probe the active site with magnetic resonance techniques. In the functioning of the ATPase, Mn^{2+} can substitute for Mg^{2+}, and Tl^+ can substitute for K^+ [34]. Since Mn^{2+} is paramagnetic, its interaction with proteins can be monitored by its ESR spectrum. It will also increase the relaxation rates of neighboring magnetically active nuclei such as water protons and Tl^+ ions and thereby broaden the lines of their NMR spectra.

It has been shown by using ESR to monitor the binding of Mn^{2+} that there is one tight binding site per 250,000 daltons [35]. The dissociation constant determined by ESR in the presence of 100 mM NaCl and 10 nM KCl corresponds to the kinetically determined value of 0.88 μM. By determining the effectiveness with which Mg^{2+} could compete for Mn^{2+} in binding to the ATPase, ESR studies give a dissociation constant of 1 mM for Mg^{2+}. The kinetically determined value is 0.9 mM. In addition to the tight divalent ion binding site, there are 200-400 looser binding sites that are probably due to binding to phospholipid in the preparation, since at saturating levels the divalent-ion-to-phosphate ratio is close to unity.

The environment of the Mn^{2+} in the Mn^{2+} enzyme can be studied by observing the effect of the Mn^{2+} on the NMR spectra of adjacent water molecules. By this method, it was found that a tight Mn^{2+}-phosphate-monovalent ion complex was formed with the enzyme in which the phosphate was probably covalently bound [35]. A stable complex is formed with phosphate monoanion and Na^+ at low pH and with phosphate dianion and K^+ at high pH.

Thallous ion, which can be studied by NMR, binds to the K^+ site and activates the ATPase at low concentrations, while at high concentrations it binds to the Na^+ site. The enzyme-bound Mn^{2+} is near the Tl^+ binding site, increasing the nuclear relaxation rate of the Tl^+ and therefore broadening its NMR line. Since the degree of broadening depends on the distance between the ions Mn^{2+} and Tl^+, it is possible to calculate it. Under conditions for which Tl^+ should be binding to the Na^+ site, the distance is 4.0 ± 0.1 Å [36]. This distance is so small that it is likely that the ions Mn^{2+} and Tl^+ are sharing a common anionic ligand, perhaps the active site aspartate. A crystallographic study of $Tl_2Mn_2(SO_4)_3$ has shown that when Mn^{2+} and Tl^+ share a common oxygen, the distance is 3.89 Å [37]. With two ions in such close proximity, it would be expected that owing to electrostatic effects, the binding of one ion would increase the dissociation constant of the other ion. Supporting this, the dissociation constant for Mg^{2+} is increased from 0.15 mM to 1 mM by the addition of 100 mM NaCl and 10 mM KCl. Furthermore, Tl^+ and Mn^{2+} mutually increase their K_m values for activation of the ATPase. Extrapolation to zero-free Mn^{2+} gives a K_m for Tl^+ of 0.03 mM, and for extrapolation to infinite-free Mn^{2+}, the K_m for Tl^+ is 0.56 mM. For zero Tl^+ concentration, the K_m for Mn^{2+} is 0.26 μM, and for infinite Tl^+ the K_m is 2.6 μM [36]. The binding of phosphate perturbs the Mn^{2+}-to-Tl^+ distance, increasing it to 5.4 Å. This distance is consistent with Mn^{2+} and Tl^+ as ligands of different oxygen atoms of the same phosphate group. The simplest interpretation of the results is that in the absence of phosphate, Mn^{2+} and Tl^+ have as a common ligand the aspartate carboxylate oxygen in the enzyme-active site. On addition of phosphate, the phosphate phosphorylates the aspartate, with the ions Mn^{2+} and Tl^+ becoming ligands of different oxygens of the phosphate group of the acyl phosphate. A model for the active site of the ATPase is shown in Figure 1.

In the presence of a divalent metal ion, the Na^+-K^+ ATPase catalyzes a rapid exchange of ^{18}O between water and phosphate [38, 39]. The exchange is inhibited by Na^+ and stimulated by K^+. Ouabain, which inhibits the ATPase, also inhibits the exchange reaction. Analysis of the ^{18}O exchange data shows that the acyl phosphate intermediate hydrolyzes by P–O bond cleavage rather than C–O bond cleavage. This implies that the phosphorylation of the ATPase by phosphate proceeds by direct attack of the carboxylate oxygen on phosphate ion, and that in hydrolysis of the acyl phosphate water attacks the phosphate phosphorus rather than acyl group carbonyl.

Another important aspect of the mechanism of the Na^+-K^+ ATPase is its inhibition by cardiac glycosides. The ATPase is the putative receptor for the ionotropic effects of cardiac glycosides on the heart [40, 41]. The glycoside that has been most extensively studied is ouabain. Ouabain binding is slow, with the kinetics of binding and inhibition identical [42]. The rate of binding is a complex function of nucleotide, monovalent ion, divalent ion, and phosphate concentrations [42, 43]. Both the rate and the equilibrium constant for binding depend on the tissue and species source [44, 45]. The aglycone is also a potent inhibitor [46]. The initial kinetic studies indicated that the stimulating effect of Na^+ and the inhibitory effect of K^+ on ouabain binding could be explained by a mechanism in which ouabain bound only to E_2 – P [42]. Supporting this interpretation, it has been found that ouabain has little effect on dephosphorylation of $E_1 \sim P$, while dephosphorylation of E_2 – P is strongly inhibited [25]. This analysis of ouabain binding is somewhat oversimplified, however, since ouabain binding can occur in the absence of phosphorylation [47], dephosphorylation of E_2 – P in the presence of K^+ is not inhibited [25], and there is kinetic evidence for two types of ouabain binding sites [43].

The purified Na^+-K^+ ATPase, regardless of the method of purification, has considerable bound phospholipid [17–21, 48], which in those cases in

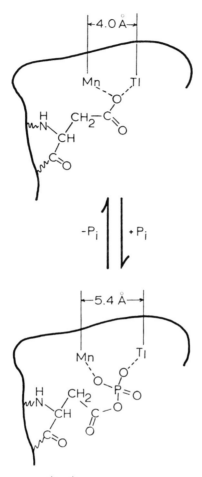

FIG. 1 A model for the Na$^+$- K$^+$ ATPase active site based on NMR and
ESR active site probes.

which it was examined behaves as a phospholipid bilayer [19, 48]. Electron
micrographs of the purified enzyme appear as membrane vesicles [20]. During
purification, there is no dramatic change in lipid composition (Table 2), although more detailed analysis may show differences in phospholipid head
groups and fatty acid side chains. There may be changes in lipid organization
on purification but contradictory results are obtained, depending on the technique used [49, 50]. For example, steroid spin labels indicate greater organization, while fatty acid ester labels suggest greater fluidity. Detergents used
in the purification of the ATPase can dramatically reduce the turnover number, possibly by affecting lipid structure [18, 20].

TABLE 2

Lipid Analyses on Kidney Medulla Plasma Membranes
and Purified Na^+-K^+ ATPase[a]

	Plasma membrane	Na^+-K^+ ATPase
Protein/lipid (2/2)	3.8	1.72
% Cholesterol[b]	26	24
% Phospholipid[b]	62	57
% Noncholesterol neutral lipid[b]	12	19
Total unsaturation (μeq/mg lipid)[c]	3.85	3.54

Source: Ref. 48.

[a]Specific activity 14-18 units/mg, $\approx$40% pure.

[b]Based on total lipid.

[c]Determined by Br_2 consumption.

IV. THE ROLE OF LIPIDS

The Na^+-K^+ ATPase is inhibited by treatments known to destroy or remove lipids. Detergents [49–52], lipases [53–56], lipid oxidation [57], and solvent extraction [58] inactivate the ATPase. ATPase activity can be restored by adding back appropriate lipids. There has been considerable controversy, however, about whether specific lipids are essential for reconstitution. Various investigators have restored activity with lecithin [59], phosphatidyl ethanolamine [60], phosphatidyl serine [61–63], phosphatidyl glycerol [64, 65], esters of phosphoric acid, and long-chain alcohols [66] and cholesterol [58]. Interpretation of the results is difficult. The lipid may be functioning by removing inhibitory detergent or products of lipase action. In most instances commercial lipids were used that were probably impure. Even synthetic phospholipids may contain impurities that alter the behavior of the lipids [67]. A more serious problem with the reconstitution experiments is that the delipidation procedures may not remove all the lipid from the ATPase, with a tight boundary layer of lipid remaining with the enzyme. It is likely that a boundary layer of tightly bound lipid will be found to be a common feature of intrinsic membrane proteins [68]. Although the various reconstitution experiments have left unresolved whether any specific lipid is essential for ATPase function, they have established that it is likely that lipids are involved.

A different type of approach to the role of lipids in ATPase function is to use probe techniques to examine lipid-protein interactions. The two most commonly used techniques are fluorescence [69–71] and spin labeling [72–74].

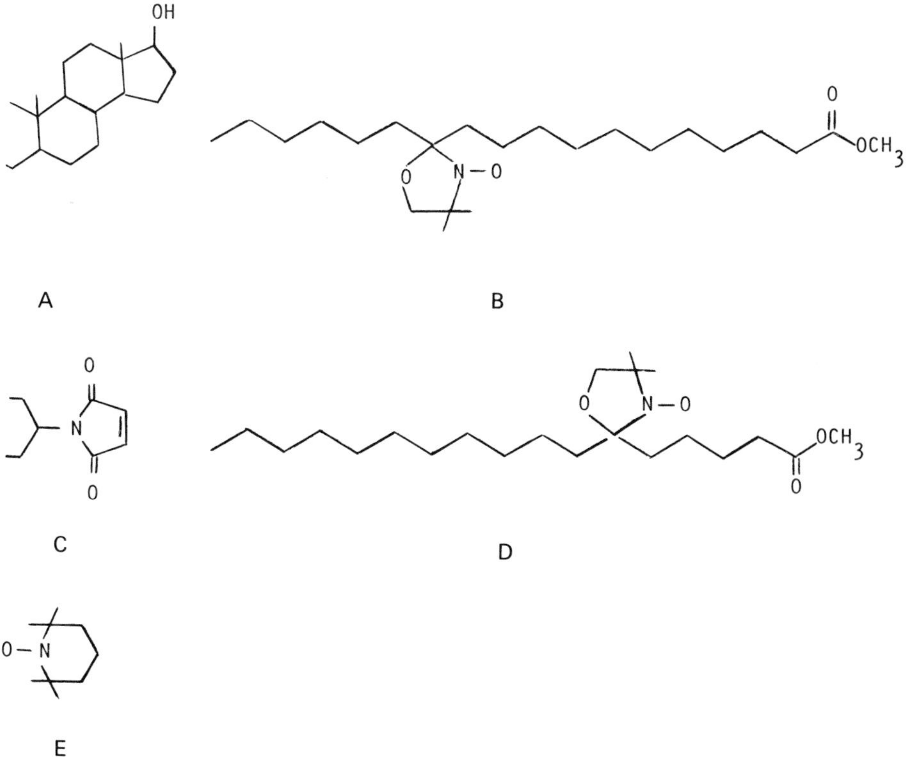

A   B

C   D

E

FIG. 2 Structure of different spin labels used in studies of the Na$^+$-K$^+$ ATPase and its interaction with lipids.

The effect of various denaturants on ATPase-lipid interactions has been examined by the spin-labeling technique [49, 75]. Lipids in association with the ATPase preparation were spin-labeled with either label (A) or label (B), and the ATPase protein had label (C). Examples of typical ESR spectra are shown in Figure 3. The ATPase preparation was active after labeling.

Adding alcohols and dioxane produced progressive changes in the ESR spectra of the lipid labels, indicating that the label became decreasingly oriented in the membrane. The alcohol concentration at which enzyme activity was irreversibly lost corresponded well with the point at which the lipid bilayer was optimally perturbed. This also depended on the alcohol, with ethanol producing a fivefold greater effect than octanol. That enzyme denaturation and a transition in lipid structure as monitored by the spin labels always occur at the same concentration of alcohol, together with absence of change in gross protein structure as monitored by the protein spin label, make it

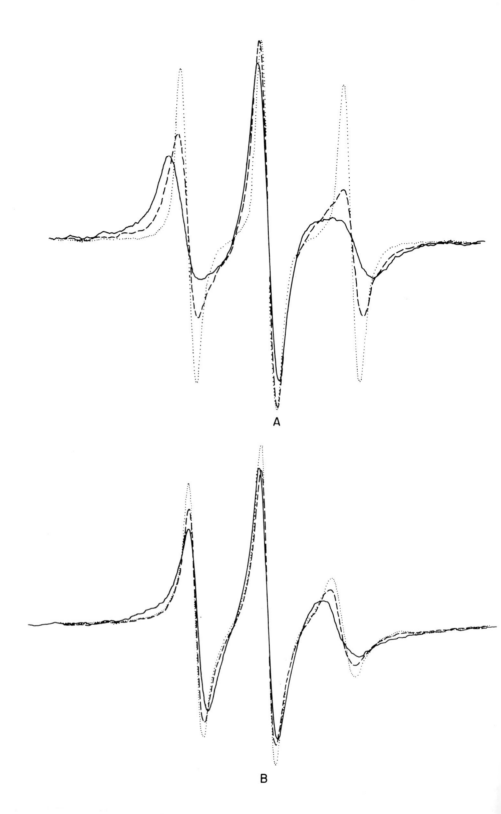

A

B

quite likely that an organized lipid structure is essential for enzyme activity. On the other hand, it is possible, by using guanidine hydrochloride, to denature the ATPase without disrupting lipid structure. Guanidine hydrochloride has little effect on the ESR spectrum of ATPase labeled with (E) until a denaturing concentration is reached; at that point, the mobility of the label dramatically increases. There is no effect on either lipid label.

More direct evidence for lipid involvement in Na$^+$-K$^+$ ATPase function comes from the thermal behavior of the enzyme. Several investigators have observed that the Arrhenius plot for ATPase activity is decidedly nonlinear [76–78]. The data appear to be best fitted by two straight lines that intersect at 20 °C. The activation energy above 20 °C is 12–16 Kcal/mole, while below 20 °C it is 30–40 Kcal/mole. If the transition from one slope to the other is occurring over a temperature range 1°–5 °C, the Van't Hoff ΔH for the process must be several hundred Kcal/mole, suggesting a highly cooperative process. Since phospholipids undergo phase transitions and phase separations, they are the most likely candidate for the cause of the anomalous temperature behavior of the ATPase. The heat of transition for the phospholipid liquid–crystal-to-gel phase transition is near 10 Kcal/mole for most

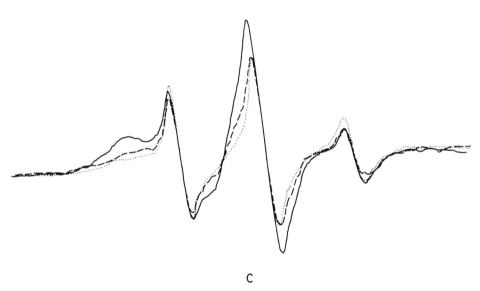

C

FIG. 3 (Left and above) A. Purified Na$^+$-K$^+$ ATPase labeled with probe A for no added ethanol (——), 22% ethanol (---), and 40% ethanol (···). B. Purified Na$^+$-K$^+$ ATPase labeled with the methyl ester of probe B for no t-butanol (——), 12% t-butanol (---), and 20% t-butanol (···). C. Purified Na$^+$-K$^+$ ATPase labeled with probe E for no added guanidine·HCl (——), 1.1 M guanidine·HCl (---), and 2 M guanidine·HCl (···).

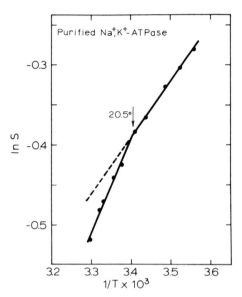

FIG. 4 Temperature dependence of S for probe D in the purified Na^+-K^+ ATPase lipids.

phospholipids [79]. In the purified ATPase preparation, the molar ratio of phospholipid to ATPase is approximately 150:1 [48]. Thus a phase transition involving only 10%–20% of the phospholipids would be sufficient to account for the change in slope in the Arrhenius plot. If we assume a three-degree range for the change in slope, the heat capacity change $\Delta C_p°$ would be 5,300 cal/mole of ATPase/deg, or 0.013 cal/gram membrane/deg. Unfortunately, this is far too small to detect calorimetrically. However, by use of the spin-labeled fatty acid methyl ester (D), it is possible to see a structural transition in the membrane lipids of the purified ATPase that occurs at 20 °C (Fig. 4). The transition can still be seen in liposomes prepared from lipids extracted from the ATPase membranes [50]. This strongly supports the supposition that the anomalous temperature behavior of the ATPase is due to a structural transition in the lipids. While the extracted lipids showed a structural transition at the same temperature as the membrane fragments, the motion of the label was less restricted, implying that the ATPase protein has an ordering effect on the lipids [50]. This is consistent with a boundary lipid model of Jost et al. [68]. It is surprising, however, that such protein-lipid interactions do not alter the transition temperature. This phenomenon has also been seen in other membrane preparations; that is, the membrane proteins have an ordering or restricting effect on the membrane lipids but little or no effect on the transition temperature [80].

Similar conclusions have been reached with a reconstituted Na^+-K^+ ATPase prepared from sodium deoxycholate-inactivated enzyme. The enzyme reconstituted with dimyristoyl-, dipalmitoyl-, distearoyl-, and dioleoyl-phosphatidyl glycerol, and bovine phosphatidyl serine showed temperature behavior that reflected the phase behavior of the lipids as studied by differential scanning calorimetry [81]. For the saturated phosphatidyl glycerols, the change in slope in the ATPase Arrhenius plot occurred 1°-8° lower than the onset of the endothermic transitions in the pure lipid. ATPase reconstituted with dioleoylphosphatidyl glycerol, which is fully melted above 0 °C, shows no change of slope in its Arrhenius plot. Bovine phosphatidyl serine shows a broad transition at 13°; the reconstituted ATPase shows a change in slope in its temperature plot at approximately 15 °C.

The nature of the structural transition occurring in the membrane lipids that affects ATPase activity has yet to be determined. The lipid transition at 20 °C can also be seen, using E (TEMPO) as a probe (Fig. 5). In this study K', the apparent partition coefficient, was determined, to facilitate comparison with pure phospholipid dispersions. From Figure 5, it can be seen that K' decreases about tenfold when dipalmitoyl phosphatidylcholine undergoes the liquid-crystal-to-gel phase transition. In the temperature range 0°-50°, K' varies from 7 to 15 for lamb kidney medulla plasma membranes. Thus even at 0 °C, TEMPO has greater solubility in the kidney membranes than in the liquid crystal state of dipalmitoyl lecithin. Furthermore, the change in K' over a 50° temperature range is quite small. It is therefore unlikely that the structural change occurring at 20 °C is a liquid-crystal-to-gel phase transition involving the bulk of the membrane lipids. Such a transition is also unlikely when one considers how highly unsaturated the membrane lipids are (Table 2). These observations suggest that the structural transition occurring at 20 °C is a separation out of a small region of a gel-like phase within the membrane, with the Na^+-K^+ ATPase located principally in that phase.

The step in the Na^+-K^+ ATPase catalytic sequence that is the most likely one to be affected by the lipid structural transition is the E_1-to-E_2 conformational change, and there is some evidence to support this hypothesis [82]. The change in slope at 20 °C in the Na^+-K^+ ATPase plot must represent a change in rate-determining step. The activation energy for phosphorylation of the ATPase by ATP is quite small, and the Arrhenius plot is linear [83]. There is a ouabain-inhibitable K^+-p-nitrophenylphosphatase activity in purified Na^+-K^+ ATPase preparations that is presumably analogous to the K^+-activated dephosphorylation of the enzyme, with p-nitrophenylphosphate rather than E_2 - P (Eq. (3)) acting as substrate.

Oligomycin, which is thought to block the conversion of $E_1 \sim P$ to E_2 - P, does not inhibit the K^+-p-nitrophenylphosphatase, and so that conversion is not part of the phosphatase action. The Arrhenius plot for the K^+-p-nitrophenylphosphatase is linear, with activation energy 8.9 Kcal/mole [82]. Thus

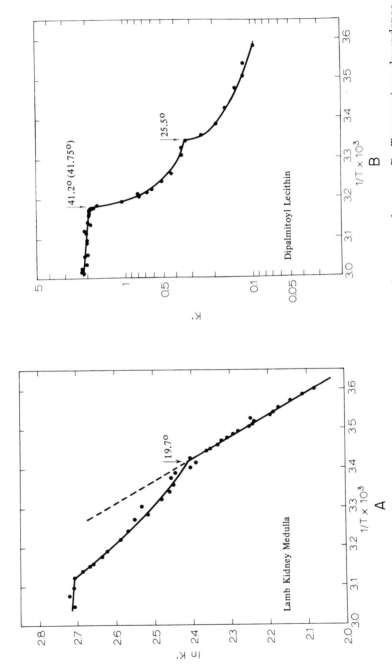

FIG. 5 Temperature dependence of K' for TEMPO in kidney plasma membranes. B. Temperature dependence of K' for TEMPO in dipalmitoyl lecithin.

the temperature dependence of the steps of Eqs. (1) and (3) are linear, with low activation energies, while the Na$^+$- K$^+$ ATPase has nonlinear Arrhenius plot, with an activation energy much larger than either the phosphorylation step or the phosphatase step, even when the lipids are in the liquid crystal state [50, 81]. This does not prove, but does make likely, that it is the E_1-to-E_2 conformational change that is affected by the lipid structural change.

V. SUMMARY

With the advent of relatively pure Na$^+$- K$^+$ ATPase preparations, it has been possible to obtain a fair amount of information about the structure and mechanism of the enzyme. This review has concentrated on information obtained from the use of NMR and ESR techniques. Concerning the active site of the enzyme, it has been found that the monovalent and divalent cation–binding sites are in close proximity, with a possible model of the active site shown in Figure 1. The studies on the role of lipids in Na$^+$- K$^+$ ATPase function have established that an organized lipid structure is required for activity. From a comparison of the effects of temperature on the ATPase and on lipid structure in the same membrane fragments, it can be concluded that although an organized lipid structure is required, the lipid component of the membrane must be in a fluid, liquid–crystalline state.

REFERENCES

1. J. L. Dahl and L. E. Hokin, Ann. Rev. Biochem., 43, 327–356 (1974).
2. A. Schwartz, G. E. Lindenmayer, and J. C. Allen, in Current Topics in Membranes and Transport, ed. F. Bonner and A. Kleinzeller, Vol. 3. New York: Academic Press, 1973, pp. 1–82.
3. P. J. Garrahan and I. M. Glynn, J. Physiol., 192, 237 (1967).
4. V. L. Lew, I. M. Glynn, and J. C. Ellory, Nature, 225, 865 (1970).
5. I. M. Glynn, Brit. Med. Bull., 24, 165 (1968).
6. P. J. Garrahan and I. M. Glynn, J. Physiol., 192, 217 (1967).
7. L. J. Mullins and F. J. Brinly, J. Gen. Physiol., 53, 704 (1969).
8. P. C. Caldwell and R. D. Keyes, J. Physiol., 148, 8P (1959).
9. J. C. Skou, Physiol. Rev., 45, 596 (1965).
10. G. R. Kepner and R. I. Macey, Biochim. Biophys. Acta, 163, 188 (1968).
11. P. K. Lauf, Ann. N.Y. Acad. Sci., 242, 324 (1974).
12. R. Blostein, P. K. Lauf, and D. C. Tosteson, Biochim. Biophys. Acta, 249, 623 (1971).
13. J. R. Sachs, Ann. N.Y. Acad. Sci., 242, 343 (1974).
14. C. H. Joiner and P. K. Lauf, Fed. Proc., 33, 265 (1974).
15. J. J. Snyder, B. A. Rasmussen, and P. K. Lauf, J. Immunol., 197, 772 (1971).

16. L. D. Frye and M. Edidin, J. Cell. Sci., 7, 319 (1970).

17. P. L. Jørgensen, J. C. Skou, and L. P. Solomonsen, Biochim. Biophys. Acta, 233, 381 (1971).

18. J. Kyte, J. Biol. Chem., 247, 7642 (1972).

19. L. E. Hokin, J. L. Dahl, J. D. Deupree, J. F. Dixon, J. F. Hackney, and J. F. Perdue, J. Biol. Chem., 248, 2593 (1973).

20. P. L. Jørgensen, Ann. N.Y. Acad. Sci., 242, 36 (1974).

21. M. Nakao, T. Nakao, Y. Hara, F. Nagai, S. Yagasaki, M. Koi, A. Nakagawa, and K. Kawai, Ann. N.Y. Acad. Sci., 242, 24 (1974).

22. K. Nagano, T. Kanazawa, N. Mizuno, Y. Tashima, T. Nakao, and M. Nakao, Biochem. Biophys. Res. Commun., 19, 759 (1965).

23. R. L. Post and S. Kume, J. Biol. Chem., 248, 6993 (1973).

24. C. Degani, A. S. Dahms, and P. D. Boyer, Ann. N.Y. Acad. Sci., 242, 77 (1974).

25. R. L. Post, G. Toda, and Faye N. Rogers, J. Biol. Chem., 250, 691 (1975).

26. S. Fahn, M. R. Hurley, G. J. Koval, and R. W. Albers, J. Biol. Chem., 241, 1890 (1966).

27. T. Tobin, A. Akera, and T. M. Brody, Ann. N.Y. Acad. Sci., 242, 120 (1974).

28. R. L. Post, S. Kume, T. Tobin, B. Orcutt, and A. K. Sen, J. Gen. Physiol., 54, 3065 (1969).

29. G. J. Siegel, G. J. Koval, and R. W. Albers, J. Biol. Chem., 244, 3264 (1969).

30. L. E. Hokin and J. L. Dahl, in Metabolic Pathways, ed. L. E. Hokin, 3rd ed., vol. 6. New York: Academic Press, 1971, p. 269.

31. R. L. Post, K. Taniguchi, and G. Toda, Ann. N.Y. Acad. Sci., 242, 80 (1974).

32. W. P. Jencks, in Handbook of Biochemistry, ed. H. Sober, J 144. Cleveland: Chemical Rubber Co., 1968.

33. R. W. Albers, Ann. Rev. Biochem., 36, 727 (1967).

34. J. S. Britten and M. Blank, Biochim. Biophys. Acta, 159, 160 (1968).

35. C. Grisham and A. Mildvan, J. Biol. Chem., 249, 3187 (1974).

36. C. M. Grisham, R. K. Gupta, R. E. Barnett, and A. S. Mildvan, J. Biol. Chem., 249, 6738 (1974).

37. A. Zemann and J. Zemann, Acta Crystallogr. Sect. B., 10, 409 (1957).

38. A. S. Dahms, T. Kanazawa, and P. D. Boyer, J. Biol. Chem., 248, 6592 (1973).

39. A. S. Dahms and P. D. Boyer, J. Biol. Chem., 248, 3155 (1973).

40. H. R. Besch, J. C. Allen, G. Glick, and A. Schwartz, J. Pharmacol. Exp. Ther., 171, 1 (1970).

41. T. Akera, F. S. Larsen, and T. M. Brody, J. Pharmacol. Exp. Ther., 174, 145 (1970).

42. R. E. Barnett, Biochemistry, 9, 4644 (1970).

43. C. Inagaki, G. E. Lindenmayer, and A. Schwartz, J. Biol. Chem., 249, 5135 (1974).

44. T. Tobin and T. M. Brody, Biochem. Pharm., 21, 1553 (1972).
45. A. Yoda, Ann. N.Y. Acad. Sci., 242, 598 (1974).
46. S. M. Kupchan, M. Mokotoff, R. S. Sandhu, and L. E. Hokin, J. Med. Chem., 10, 1025 (1967).
47. A. Schwartz, H. Matsui, and A. H. Laughter, Science, 160, 323 (1968).
48. C. M. Grisham, Ph.D. thesis, University of Minnesota (1973).
49. C. M. Grisham and R. E. Barnett, Biochim. Biophys. Acta, 266, 613 (1972).
50. C. M. Grisham and R. E. Barnett, Biochemistry, 12, 2635 (1973).
51. I. M. Glynn, Biochem. J., 84, 75P (1962).
52. J. C. Skou, Biochim. Biophys. Acta, 58, 314 (1962).
53. H. J. Portius and K. Repke, Arch. Exptl. Pathol. Pharmacol., 245, 62 (1963).
54. J. C. Skou, in Membrane Transport and Metabolism, ed. A. Kleinzeller and A. Kotyk. New York: Academic Press, 1961, p. 228.
55. J. H. Schatzmann, Nature, 196, 677 (1922).
56. M. Tatibana, J. Biochem., 53, 260 (1963).
57. I. Tateishi, M. Steiner, and M. G. Baldini, J. Lab. Clin. Med., 81, 587 (1973).
58. J. Jarnefelt, Biochim. Biophys. Acta, 266, 91 (1972).
59. R. Tanaka and K. P. Strickland, Arch. Biochem. Biophys., 111, 583 (1965).
60. K. Taniguchi and Y. Tonomura, J. Biochem., 69, 543 (1971).
61. K. P. Wheeler and R. Whittam, J. Physiol., 207, 303 (1970).
62. K. P. Wheeler and R. Whittam, Nature, 225, 449 (1970).
63. T. Ohnishi and H. Kawamura, J. Biochem., 56, 377 (1964).
64. H. K. Kimelberg and D. Papahadjopoulos, Biochim. Biophys. Acta, 232, 265 (1972).
65. P. Palatini, F. Dabbeni-Sala, and A. Bruni, Biochim. Biophys. Acta, 288, 413 (1972).
66. R. Tanaka and T. Sakamoto, Biochim. Biophys. Acta, 193, 384 (1969).
67. H. L. Kantor and J. H. Prestegard, Biochemistry, 14, 1790 (1975).
68. P. C. Jost, O. H. Griffith, R. A. Capaldi, and G. Vanderkooi, Proc. Nat. Acad. Sci., 70, 480 (1973).
69. U. Cogan, M. Shinitzky, G. Weber, and T. Nishida, Biochemistry, 12, 521 (1973).
70. M. Shinitzky and Y. Barenholz, J. Biol. Chem., 249, 2652 (1974).
71. B. Rudy and C. Gitler, Biochim. Biophys. Acta, 288, 231 (1972).
72. H. M. McConnell and B. McFarland, Quart. Rev. Biophys., 3, 91 (1970).
73. I. C. P. Smith, in Biological Applications of Electron Spin Resonance, ed. H. M. Swartz, J. R. Bolton, and D. C. Berg. New York: Wiley-Interscience, 1972, p. 483.
74. D. F. H. Wallach and R. J. Winzler, in Evolving Strategies and Tactics in Membrane Research. New York: Springer-Verlag, 1974, chap. 8.

75. C. M. Grisham and R. E. Barnett, Biochim. Biophys. Acta, 311, 417 (1973).
76. N. Gruener and Y. Avi-Dor, J. Biochem., 100, 762 (1966).
77. J. S. Charnock, D. M. Doty, and J. C. Russell, Arch. Biochem. Biophys., 142, 633 (1971).
78. J. S. Charnock, D. A. Cook, A. F. Almeida, and R. To, Arch. Biochem. Biophys., 159, 393 (1973).
79. B. D. Ladbrooke and D. Chapman, Chem. Phys. Lipids, 3, 304 (1969).
80. C. D. Linden, K. L. Wright, H. M. McConnell, and C. F. Fox, Proc. Nat. Acad. Sci., 70, 2271 (1973).
81. H. K. Kimelberg and D. Papahadjopoulos, J. Biol. Chem., 249, 1071 (1974).
82. R. E. Barnett and J. Palazzotto, Ann. N.Y. Acad. Sci., 242, 69 (1974).
83. A. H. Neufeld and H. M. Levy, J. Biol. Chem., 245, 4962 (1970).

Chapter 6

THE GLYCOPROTEINS OF THE SEMLIKI FOREST VIRUS MEMBRANE

Kai Simons
Henrik Garoff
Ari Helenius

European Molecular Biology Laboratory
Heidelberg, Federal Republic of Germany

I. INTRODUCTION

Many animal, plant, and bacterial viruses contain lipid membranes [1-4].
Some produce widespread diseases in humans (e.g., smallpox, yellow fever,
influenza, measles, parotitis, and encephalitis), and membrane viruses have
therefore long been intensively studied in medical virology departments.
More recently, membrane viruses have been used by molecular biologists to
probe into host cell structure and function. In this review, we shall focus on

one such virus, the Semliki Forest virus (SFV). This virus is one of the simplest among the membrane viruses. Semliki Forest virus contains a spherical nucleocapsid (diameter 40 nm) [7], which is composed of one single-stranded RNA molecule (molecular weight 4.5×10^6) [8] and one lysine-rich protein species, the nucleocapsid protein [9]. The nucleocapsid is covered by a lipid membrane (cross section 4.5 nm) that is studded by glycoprotein surface projections 7.5 nm long [10].

The Semliki Forest virus is a member of the alphaviruses of the togavirus family (this virus group was formerly known as the arbo A group). The alphaviruses are spread by blood-sucking arthropods (mainly mosquitoes) in nature and have a wide host range [5–6]. These viruses can be grown in avian, mammalian, or insect cells in culture and they grow well over a wide range of temperatures [25 °C–41 °C]. This probably reflects their natural adaptation both to poikilothermic and to homeothermic organisms. However, vertebrate and invertebrate cells differ in their modes of alphavirus replication. In vertebrate cells, alphavirus infection is cytopathic; host RNA and protein synthesis stop within a few hours after infection [11–12]. The nucleocapsids are assembled in the cytoplasm of the host cell, and attach to the cytoplasmic surface of the plasma membrane. The nucleocapsids then bud out of the cell through the membrane into the extracellular fluid and are thereby enveloped by a modified segment of the host cell plasma membrane [13]. In invertebrate cells, on the other hand, the virus infection is much less toxic to the cell. Infected cells grow and divide normally for many generations [14]. Electron-microscopic studies have shown that in these cells virus replication and maturation take place inside cytoplasmic vesicles [15]. The vesicles contain ribosomes and complex laminate membrane structures reminiscent of the Golgi apparatus. When the viruses are completed, the entire content of the vesicle is released into the extracellular fluid [15]. Little is yet known of the molecular events of SFV replication in the insect cells. Most studies on SFV have been done using avian or mammalian cells as hosts. In our laboratory we have mainly used baby hamster kidney cells (BHK21), in which the virus grows to high titers.

II. SOLUBILIZATION AND ISOLATION OF THE SFV MEMBRANE PROTEINS

The SFV membrane contains lipids and proteins in a weight ratio of about 2 : 3 [16]. The membrane lipids are derived from the host cell plasma membrane, and the viral lipid composition is different depending on the host cell used [17–19]. The most dramatic differences have been documented by Renkonen et al., who have found that SFV grown in baby hamster kidney (BHK21) cells and in insect (Aedes albopictus) cells have only about 36% of their phospholipids in common [20].

In contrast to the lipids, all the proteins in the virus membrane are virus-specified [21]. Three polypeptides are found in the SFV membrane: E1, E2, and E3 [22]. The proteins form spikes projecting from the external surface of the virus particle [23-24]. The spikes bind to receptor structures on the host cell surface and facilitate the passage of the viral nucleic acid into the cell. The virus receptors present on erythrocytes can be used as a convenient hemagglutination assay for the virus spike proteins [25].

The SFV membrane spike proteins are intrinsic (integral) membrane proteins; that is, they can be extracted from the membrane only by disrupting the membrane with detergents or organic solvents. Such proteins are usually amphiphilic in their structure, having a polar surface facing the aqueous exterior and an apolar part inside the hydrocarbon region of the lipid bilayer membrane (see Section III D). The proteins are thus adapted to a location in the interphase between hydrocarbon and water. If the interphase is destroyed, for instance by the use of organic solvents, the conformations of the proteins are usually severely disrupted or the proteins precipitate. Detergents can be used to circumvent the problems of denaturation and insolubility, and they seem to provide the only generally useful method for the solubilization of amphiphilic membrane proteins. We have recently dealt with this subject in a general review [26], and we shall here specifically describe the interactions of sodium dodecyl sulfate (SDS), Triton X-100, and sodium deoxycholate (DOC) with the SFV membrane. The breakdown of the virus was induced by a stepwise increase of the detergent concentration and the solubilization process was followed, using analytical ultracentrifugation, sucrose density gradient centrifugation, and electron microscopy. Detergent binding to the virus was measured, using radioactively labeled detergent under equilibrium conditions. For the detailed methodology, the reader is referred to Ref. 27 for SDS, to Refs. 28 and 29 for Triton X-100, and to Ref. 30 for DOC.

A. Solubilization with Sodium Dodecyl Sulfate

Sodium dodecyl sulfate binds with high affinity to the viral membrane (see binding isotherm in Figure 1). At free-equilibrium SDS concentrations of about 5×10^{-5} M (when 4,000-5,000 molecules of SDS are bound per virus), lysis of the viral membranes begins. The virus membrane itself contains 1.6×10^4 cholesterol molecules, and 1.8×10^4 phospholipid molecules. Lysis of the viral membrane coincides with a rapid cooperative increase in SDS binding (Fig. 1) which may be due to the sudden accessibility of the internal membrane surface and perhaps to the loss of restraints on membrane volume. Dissociation of the nucleocapsid into RNA and protein takes place already at free SDS concentrations below 1×10^{-4} M. At successively higher SDS concentrations, solubilization of the membrane into lipoprotein complexes occurs; these decrease in size and lipid content, and finally separate protein-SDS complexes and lipid-SDS mixed micelles are obtained. Free SDS

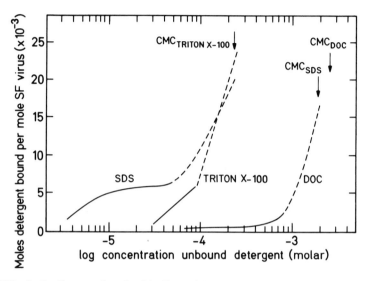

FIG. 1 Isotherms for the binding of SDS, DOC, and Triton X-100 to SFV. The SDS and the Triton X-100 isotherms were done at 4 °C, whereas the DOC isotherm was done at 20 °C. Taken from Refs. 27 and 30.

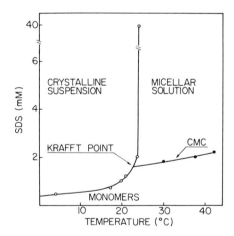

FIG. 2 Temperature-concentration phase diagram of SDS in 0.1 M NaCl/0.05 M sodium phosphate, pH 7.4. CMC, critical micellar concentration. At low temperatures the detergent forms insoluble crystals. The monomer concentration in equilibrium with the crystals is below the CMC until the Krafft point is reached, at which micelles begin to form. Taken from Ref. 27.

concentrations of 0.75×10^{-3} M are sufficient for complete delipidation (at 30 °C), indicating that the whole sequence from lysis to delipidation occurs at SDS concentrations below the critical micellar concentration. Pure SDS micelles are therefore no prerequisite for either the solubilization or the delipidation of the membrane. The degree of virus breakdown depends basically on the amount of detergent bound per unit weight of membrane. The detergent bound to the membrane (or to its breakdown products) is in equilibrium with the free monomeric detergent, the concentration of which increases as binding increases. Therefore a reduction of the free-equilibrium detergent concentration, for instance by dialysis or dilution, results after equilibration in decreased amounts of bound detergent, which leads to the reassociation of solubilized membranes [26]. With SDS, the solubility of the free monomers depends on the temperature (see temperature-concentration phase diagram, Figure 2). At low temperatures, the reduced solubility of monomeric SDS should, according to this reasoning, reduce the amount of SDS that can be bound to membranes and this in turn could halt the membrane dissociation at some stage before delipidation. Such an effect was actually observed with SFV: at 4 °C (even in the presence of a large excess of SDS) the viruses could be lysed but not solubilized. At 20 °C they could be solubilized but not delipidated. To obtain delipidation, temperatures above the Krafft point (see Fig. 2) were needed. The temperature not only affects the solubility of SDS but probably also affects the affinity of the membrane for SDS. For instance, higher monomer concentrations were needed at 4 °C to cause lysis than at 20 °C. This effect may be mediated by changes in the properties of the lipid bilayer. It should be noted that the phase diagram (Fig. 1) is for repeatedly crystallized SDS. Commercial SDS preparations are as a rule impure and have a higher monomer solubility and a lower Krafft point [31].

When dissociation of the virus membrane by SDS was allowed to proceed to delipidation, the proteins were denatured and dissociated into their constituent polypeptide chains, and the hemagglutinating activity of the spike proteins was lost. The membrane polypeptides E1, E2, and E3 could be separated from each other in polyacrylamide gel electrophoresis in the presence of the detergent using a discontinuous buffer system (Fig. 3). Isolation of the three membrane polypeptides in milligram amounts was achieved by using chromatography on hydroxylapatite in the presence of SDS (Fig. 4). This seems to be a generally useful method for isolating SDS-polypeptide complexes [32]. Not only does the method have the advantage of being more convenient for preparative purposes than SDS-polyacrylamide gel electrophoresis but it also makes the separation of equally sized polypeptides possible. The chromatography has to be performed above the Krafft point of the SDS preparation used in order to avoid precipitation of the detergent in the column. We used a temperature of 28 °C for chromatography of the SFV proteins.

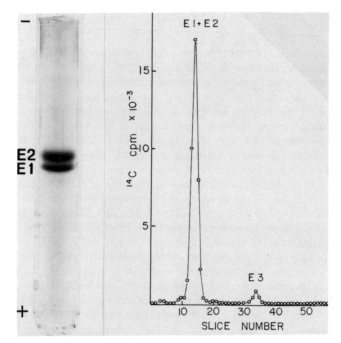

FIG. 3 SDS-polyacrylamide gel electrophoresis of the SFV membrane proteins. Left. Discontinuous system [108]. Pattern stained with Coomassic blue. E1 and E2 are stained, whereas E3 is not, presumably due to its small size and high carbohydrate content. Right. Continuous system [109]. SFV membrane proteins labeled with ^{14}C amino acids. E1 and E2 are not resolved from each other in this electrophoresis system.

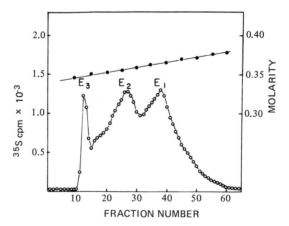

FIG. 4 Elution pattern of 4 mg delipidated SFV membrane protein, containing ^{35}S methionine, from an SDS-hydroxylapatite column (1.0×30 cm) when chromatographed with a 200-ml linear gradient of 0.3 M sodium phosphate–0.1% SDS–1 mM dithiothreitol to 0.45 M sodium phosphate–0.1% SDS–1 mM dithiothreitol. ^{35}S radioactivity (o—o); molarity of phosphate in the eluate (●—●). Taken from Ref. 22.

B. Solubilization with Triton X-100

If the mild non-ionic detergent Triton X-100 is used instead of SDS, solubilization of the SFV particle proceeds through similar stages. These are shown in the electron micrographs in Figure 5. Binding of Triton X-100 to SFV begins below the critical micellar concentration. At a free Triton X-100 concentration of 1×10^{-4} M, when more than 5,000 Triton X-100 molecules are bound to the particle, lysis of the membrane starts (Fig. 5) and the released nucleocapsid and the membrane "ghosts" can be separated by density gradient centrifugation. The nucleocapsid structure remains intact throughout the solubilization, in contrast to what was found with SDS. When the detergent concentration is increased beyond that needed for lysis, the membranes are solubilized into well-defined homogeneous lipoprotein complexes that have a diameter about 25 nm (Fig. 5). These lipoprotein complexes are finally delipidated to form separate lipid and protein Triton X-100 complexes (Fig. 6). The lipid-free protein-detergent complexes have a sedimentation coefficient of 4.5 S and a molecular weight of 1.5×10^5. They contain one molecule of E1, E2, and E3 each and in addition about 75 molecules of Triton X-100 (Table 1). This trimer probably corresponds to a spike on the virus surface (see Section IIIE) and it does not dissociate into its constituent polypeptide chains in the presence of Triton X-100 under the conditions we have tried. The SFV 4.5 S complexes aggregate readily to form a 23.5 S complex containing 260 molecules of Triton X-100 and 8 molecules of E1, E2, and E3 each (Table 1). The hemagglutinating activity associated with the spike is preserved at all stages. The aggregation of 4.5 S to 23.5 S is inhibited by sucrose, concentrations above 10% stabilizing the 4.5 S form. As the association of the 4.5 S form to the 23.5 S complex seems to proceed in almost all-or-none fashion, one can assume that there is a cooperative interaction between the associating subunits in the formation of the 23.5 S complex.

TABLE 1

Properties of the Delipidated SFV Membrane Glycoprotein Complexes Obtained with Triton X-100

	4.5 S	23.5 S	29.1 S
Stokes radius (Å)	53	94	80
$S_{20,W}$	4.5	23.5	29.1
Molecular weight	1.5×10^5	1.1×10^6	9×10^5
Polypeptide composition	$(E_1E_2E_3)$	$8(E_1E_2E_3)$	$8(E_1E_2E_3)$
Triton X-100/protein (w/w)	0.5	0.2	0.02

Source: Refs. 29 and 105.

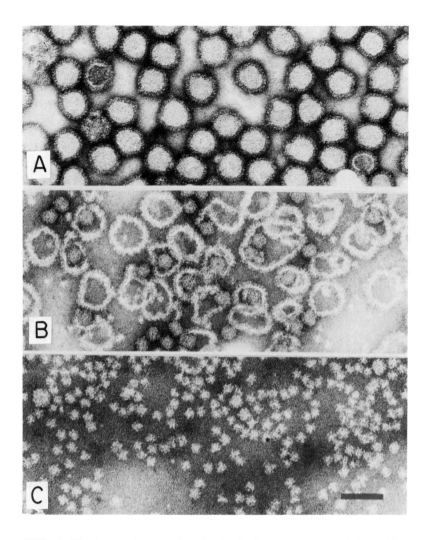

FIG. 5 Electron micrographs obtained after negative staining with potassium phosphotungstate. A. Control SFV. B. SFV treated with enough Triton X-100 to cause lysis (210 μg SFV protein and 45 μg Triton X-100 in 0.1 ml). The round 40-nm particles are the nucleocapsids. C. Lipoprotein-detergent complexes obtained from the SFV membrane when solubilized with 100 μg Triton X-100 per 100 μg SFV protein. The bar is 100 nm; all the pictures have the same magnification.

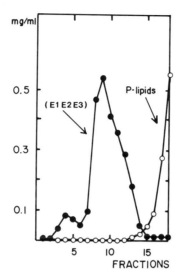

FIG. 6 Delipidation of the SFV membrane proteins with Triton X-100.
Four mg of Triton X-100 was added to SFV (1 mg protein) before application
to a 15%–25% sucrose density gradient. The gradient contained 0.05% Triton
X-100, 0.1 M NaCl, and 0.05 M Tris, pH 7.4. Sedimentation to the left.
Spinco SW50 rotor. 42,000 rpm for 24 hr at 4 °C. Taken from Ref. 29.

About 340 molecules of Triton X-100 are released from the protein–detergent
complexes when eight 4.5 S units associate to form one 23.5 S oligomer.

The SFV membrane proteins can be isolated in a monodisperse and
water–soluble form virtually free from lipid and detergent. This is done by
adding enough Triton X-100 to the virus to dissociate the lipids from the
membrane protein. The mixture is sedimented through a zone of Triton
X-100 into a detergent-free sucrose gradient (Fig. 7). The lipids stay in the
Triton zone, the nucleocapsids sediment to the bottom of the tube, and the
spike proteins are recovered as a homogeneous complex in the middle of the
gradient. The membrane protein complexes obtained have a sedimentation
coefficient of 29.1 S and a molecular weight of 9×10^5, and they contain 8
copies of E1, E2, and E3 each (Table 1). This water–soluble preparation is
virtually free from lipid and detergent and is stable for weeks at 4 °C. Since
the spike proteins of the membrane viruses carry the antigenic determinants
responsible for host immunity to viral infection, this type of a spike protein
preparation appears a promising candidate for a protein subunit vaccine.
This preparation may also be suitable for more detailed structural studies.
In electron micrographs, the 29.1 S complexes can sometimes be seen to
form paracrystalline arrays (Fig. 8B).

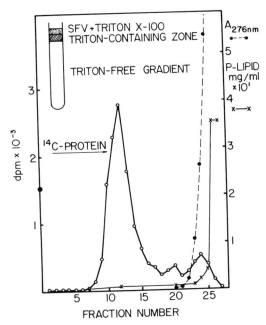

FIG. 7 Preparation of an SFV membrane protein complex virtually free of lipids and detergent. The quantity 20 mg Triton X-100 was added to SFV (1 mg protein) labeled with ^{14}C amino acids in 300 μl of 0.05 M Tris (pH 7.4)-0.1 M NaCl. The virus was layered on a 12-ml sucrose gradient (20%-50% in the same buffer) with a 0.3-ml layer of Triton X-100 in 15% sucrose on the top and centrifuged at 195,000 g for 22 hours at 20 °C. Taken from Ref. 105.

C. Solubilization with Sodium Deoxycholate

The dissociation of SFV with sodium deoxycholate (DOC) can be divided roughly into stages similar to those observed with SDS and with Triton X-100 (Table 2). The main difference is that about tenfold higher free concentrations of DOC are needed to cause lysis, solubilization, and delipidation. Prelytic binding takes place below free DOC concentrations of 0.8×10^{-3} M, and lysis of the viral membrane begins when about 2,000 molecules of DOC are bound per virus particle (Fig. 1). The effects of DOC are highly dependent on the external conditions: ionic strength, pH, and temperature. When the molarity of the sodium chloride in the 0.05 M phosphate buffer used to obtain the binding isotherm shown in Figure 1 was increased from 0.1 to 0.5 M, enough detergent was bound to cause lysis already at a free DOC concentration of 0.4×10^{-3} M. The increased detergent binding obtained at

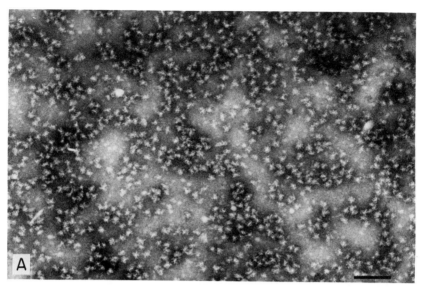

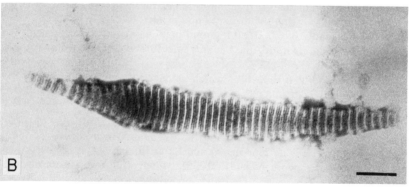

FIG. 8 Electron micrographs obtained after negative staining with potassium phosphotungstate of the (A) lipid-free and (B) detergent-free SFV membrane protein. (A. Courtesy of Dr. J. Kartenbeck. Bar 100 nm. B. Bar 100 nm.)

TABLE 2

Effects of DOC on SFV

Free DOC concentration (mM)	Effect
0 -0.8	Prelytic binding
0.8-1.5	Lysis
1.5-2.3	Solubilization and delipidation
<2.3	Dissociation of spike proteins into constituent polypeptides

higher ionic strength partly explains the well-known enhancement of the membrane solubilization efficiency of DOC with increasing salt concentrations [33]. When the pH is lowered to values approaching the pK_a, the acid form of the bile salt is formed, which is insoluble in water. The pK_a of DOC is 6.9, and at a pH of about 7.5 at room temperature DOC forms a gel. At 4 °C, DOC should be used at pH values of 8.2 or higher.

Solubilization of the viral membrane begins at 1.5×10^{-3} M. The fate of the nucleocapsids during solubilization depended on the conditions. Intact nucleocapsids could be obtained in some instances, but they frequently contained bound spike proteins and became unstable at DOC concentrations above about 2×10^{-3} M.

In contrast to Triton X-100, which released the protein spikes with its subunit structure intact, DOC dissociated the spikes at concentrations above 2.3×10^{-3} M. E1, E2, and E3 could be separated from each other at 5×10^{-3} M DOC by sucrose density gradient centrifugation (Fig. 9) or by gel filtration. E1 (and E3) were monomeric, whereas E2 was in an octamer form. Why E1 occurs as monomers and E2 as an aggregate in DOC is not clear, but this arrangement facilitates the separation of polypeptides of equal size (see Section IIIA). Both contained bound detergent, and precipitated when DOC was removed. Although DOC dissociated the spike subunit structure, the polypeptide conformation was not so drastically altered as with SDS, which caused the loss of biological activity of the polypeptides. E1 was found to be responsible for the hemagglutinating activity of the spike, whereas E2 and E3 had no such activity.

It is apparent from these studies that the sequence of events (prelytic binding, lysis, solubilization, and delipidation) was similar whether SDS, Triton X-100, or DOC was used for solubilization. The chief dissimilarity in the action of different types of detergents appears to lie in their effects on the proteins. Sodium dodecyl sulfate is generally known to be a protein denaturant [34], whereas both Triton X-100 and DOC are milder in action [35-36]. The differences between Triton X-100 and DOC can, however, be dramatic (Figs. 6 and 9). The former detergent solubilizes the spike protein

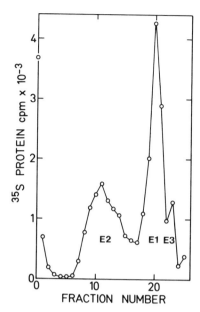

FIG. 9 Isolation of the SFV membrane proteins by sucrose density centrifugation in 13 ml 10 -50% sucrose in 100 mM NaCl, 50 mM sodium phosphate, pH 8, and 7.5 mM DOC. Sample: SFV (100 μg protein) in 0.2 ml gradient buffer. Centrifugation at 195,000 g for 16 hr at 20 °C. Taken from Ref. 30.

with its subunit structure intact and the latter dissociates the spike into its polypeptide chain constituents but with hemagglutinating activity preserved.

III. PROPERTIES OF THE SFV MEMBRANE POLYPEPTIDES

A. Molecular Weight

The molecular weight of polypeptide E3 was found to be 1×10^4, as calculated from its chemical composition [22]. The polypeptides E1 and E2 had apparent molecular weights of 4.9×10^4 and 5.2×10^4, respectively, as determined by SDS-gel electrophoresis [22]. It is assumed, however, that these proteins bind the same amount of SDS as the reference proteins (1.4 g SDS per g protein [37]). Recent studies have shown that the intrinsic membrane proteins may differ from ordinary water-soluble proteins in their SDS-binding properies [38–39]. Glycophorin (the MN-glycoprotein) of the red-blood-cell membrane appears to bind as much as 5-7 g SDS per g protein [40]. The use of SDS-gel electrophoresis for determining molecular weight may thus not be a

TABLE 3

Amino Acid Composition of SFV Membrane Glycoproteins

Amino acid	E_1	E_2	E_3
Lysine	63.6	52.0	19.9
Histidine	33.8	45.8	21.6
Arginine	36.2	48.7	60.2
Aspartic acid	88.0	84.8	114.9
Threonine	81.3	76.7	72.2
Serine	81.1	58.1	33.2
Glutamic acid	79.8	94.0	92.2
Proline	63.2	69.1	76.3
Glycine	76.3	75.1	57.3
Alanine	87.4	86.7	115.7
Half.cystine	29.3	32.1	67.6
Valine	89.2	78.2	57.1
Methionine	17.1	20.0	21.6
Isoleucine	37.5	54.4	21.7
Leucine	58.0	59.9	95.8
Tyrosine	41.0	36.4	39.5
Phenylalanine	37.2	28.0	33.2

Source: Ref. 22.
Note: Figures represent moles per 1,000 moles.

TABLE 4

Carbohydrate Composition of SFV Glycoproteins
(moles carbohydrate/mole protein)

	E1	E2	E3
N–acetylglucosamine	7	8	9
Mannose	5	12	4
Galactose	3	3	4
Fucose	1	1	2
Sialic acid	2	4	3
Total carbohydrate, % by weight	7.5%	11.5%	45.1%

Source: Ref. 22.

reliable procedure for membrane polypeptides and may yield grossly errone-
ous results. If the hydrophilic part of an amphiphilic protein is large compared with the hydrophobic part (as for E1 and E2, see Section IIID), the
molecular weights obtained may be more correct. Methods are now available,
however, for rigorous determination of molecular weights of proteins in
detergent solution (see Ref. 41).

B. Amino Acid Composition

The amino acid compositions of purified E1, E2, and E3 are shown in
Table 3. The polarity indexes calculated as described by Capaldi and Vanderkooi [42] were 0.46 for E1, 0.46 for E2, and 0.41 for E3. These proteins
are thus in the same range in hydrophobicity as water-soluble globular
proteins.

C. Carbohydrate Composition

All the SFV membrane polypeptides contain covalently linked carbohydrates.
E1 has 7.5% carbohydrate; E2, 11.5%; and E3, 45.1% (Table 4). The insolubility of the proteins is a problem in determining the carbohydrate composition. Detergents, which may affect the analysis, must be present to keep
the proteins in solution during hydrolysis. For the analysis of both neutral
monosaccharide and sialic acid content, cetyltrimethyl-ammonium bromide
was found to be better than SDS [22].

The oligosaccharide chain of E1, isolated after pronase digestion, had
a molecular weight of 3,400 and it consisted of N-acetylglucosamine, mannose, galactose, fucose, and sialic acid. E3 also had one similar carbohydrate side chain with molecular weight about 4,000, whereas E2 had one
side chain of the complex compositional type (molecular weight about 3,100)
and in addition another carbohydrate unit with molecular weight about 2,000,
containing only N-acetylglycosamine and mannose [43, cf. 44].

Schlesinger and coworkers have demonstrated an interesting application
of the membrane viruses to characterize defects in the glycosylating machinery of host cells [45]. As the glycosylation of the viral spike proteins appears
to be performed by host cell enzymes, the viral glycoproteins may be used
to pick up the oligosaccharide alterations caused by any enzymatic defect.
The advantage of this approach is that in contrast to the complexity of host
cell glycoprotein composition, the membrane viruses have only a few well-
characterized (easily purified) glycoproteins in which even subtle changes
can be detected. When Sindbis virus, a close relative of SFV, was grown in
a line (termed 15B) of Chinese hamster ovary (CHO) cells, deficient in a
specific UDP N-acetylglucosamine—glycoprotein N-acetylglucosaminyl-
transferase, virus was produced in which abnormal glycoproteins with
incomplete oligosaccharide units were present. Also, Moyer and Summers

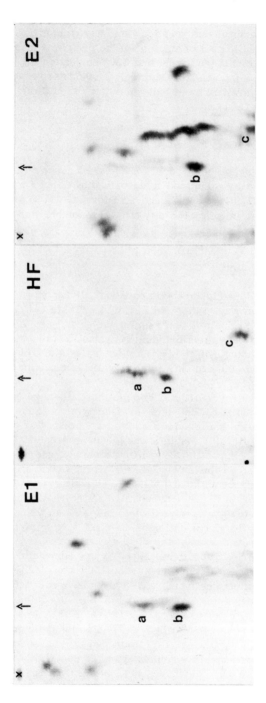

FIG. 10 Autoradiograms of two-dimensional peptide maps of E1, of E2, and of the hydrophobic peptide segment (HF). These were labeled with ^{14}C phenylalanine and digested with thermolysin. The origin is marked X. Chromatography is downward and electrophoresis to the right. ^{14}C-labeled amino acids were used as markers in the electrophoresis step and the arrow indicates the position of the neutral amino acids. Three radio-active spots marked a, b, and c were seen in the peptide map of HF. Spot b corresponds to free phenylalanine and is found in the maps of both E1 and E2. Peptide a was derived from E1 and peptide c from E2. Taken from Ref. 47.

have shown that such an approach can be used to detect and characterize small alterations in oligosaccharide structure induced by polyoma transformation of BHK cells [46].

D. Amphiphilic Properties

1. Proteolytic Digestion

When SFV is treated with the proteolytic enzyme thermolysin, all three membrane polypeptides (E1, E2, and E3) (including their oligosaccharide side chains) are cleaved off, leaving virus particles without spikes but otherwise intact [24, 47]. However, peptide segments representing about 10% of the membrane proteins are left in the membrane. These peptides are hydrophobic. The polarity index calculated from the amino acid composition is as low as 28.0, which is even lower than a similar index for brain proteolipids. Furthermore, these peptides, like phospholipids, are soluble in chloroform-methanol. The intact spike glycoproteins are not soluble in this solvent, probably because of their large hydrophilic parts.

Numerous other intrinsic membrane proteins have been shown to have similar hydrophobic peptide segments. These include cytochrome b5 [48-49] and cytochrome b5 reductase [39] in the endoplasmic reticulum, glycoprotein [50], influenza virus spike glycoproteins [51], vesicular stomatitis virus spike glycoproteins [52], filamentous phage coat protein [53], amino peptidase [54], and the sucrose-isomaltase complex [55] in the brush border membrane of the small intestine.

Peptide mapping was used to find out which of the envelope polypeptides of SFV have hydrophobic peptide tails [47]. As shown in Figure 10, both E1 and E2 were found to have their own distinct hydrophobic segments. Some technical comments may be helpful, since peptide mapping of intrinsic membrane proteins is difficult, owing to solubility problems [56]. Preferably only trace amounts of the polypeptides should be used and for this reason the proteins should be labeled with a sensitive label. If internal labeling with radioactive precursors during biosynthesis is difficult, then external labeling can be tried, using reagents specific for certain amino acids, like I^{125} or diazotized S^{35} sulfanilic acid [57]. The labeled polypeptides can be most conveniently isolated by SDS-gel electrophoresis. SDS should be removed before proteolytic digestion. The method we have found most useful for this purpose is that Weber and Kuter have described [58]. A carrier protein (e.g., albumin) should be added before this procedure to minimize losses during manipulation. Digestion is performed with fairly high concentrations of proteolytic enzymes to ensure complete cleavage of the membrane polypeptides. This is also enhanced by using enzymes with fairly wide specificity—like thermolysin, or mixtures of trypsin and chymotrypsin. Autoradiography of the peptide maps may be considerably speeded up and enhanced by fluorography [59].

It is necessary to emphasize that proteolysis is not only a valuable tool for defining membrane protein structure but also a serious cause of artifacts during membrane isolation and membrane protein purification. Almost everyone working with membrane proteins can attest to difficulties due to proteolysis by cellular enzymes. The most dramatic demonstration of how membrane proteins (especially in the presence of detergents) are prone to proteolytic degradation was the finding of miniproteins with molecular weights of less than 1×10^4 in many cellular membranes [60]. These were later shown to be proteolytic artifacts [61], some possibly deriving from hydrophobic peptide segments of intrinsic membrane proteins. The proteolytic enzymes involved in membrane-protein degradation have not yet been identified and there are no universal inhibitors available to prevent protease action. Also, purified membrane viruses contain trace amounts of proteolytic enzymes [62], but proteolysis can be minimized by working strictly in the cold, or when denaturation of the proteins is not a problem, by boiling the proteins in SDS.

2. Triton X-100 Binding

Another indication of the amphiphilic nature of the SFV spike glycoproteins is their ability to bind large amounts of Triton X-100 when delipidated. This appears to be a general property of intrinsic membrane proteins,

TABLE 5

Binding of Triton X-100 to Intrinsic Membrane Proteins

Protein	Triton X-100/protein		Reference
	W/W	Moles/complex	
Erythrocyte membrane proteins	0.2	...	35
Plasma low-density lipoprotein	0.5	...	35
Cholinergic receptor protein	0.3	...	100
Semliki Forest virus spike glycoprotein			
4.5 S complex	0.5	75	29
23.5 S complex	0.2	260	29
Cytochrome oxidase	0.3	...	101
ATPase (sarcoplasmic reticulum)	0.6	90–100	102
Rhodopsin	1.5	100	103
Cytochrome b_5	4.0	100	63
(Na^+-K^+) ATPase	0.3	60	104
Glycophorin	1.1	50	104
Erythrocyte membrane minor glycoprotein	0.8	210	104

whereas ordinary water-soluble proteins bind very little if any Triton X-100
(Table 5). Sodium deoxycholate also binds selectively to intrinsic membrane
proteins but the denaturing detergent SDS binds to all classes of proteins.
The mild detergents Triton X-100 and DOC have been shown to bind only to
the hydrophobic regions of the intrinsic membrane proteins [47, 63]. During
delipidation, the lipids around the hydrophobic regions of the protein in the
membrane are exchanged for detergents. The detergent molecules form a
micelle-like structure, which covers the apolar surface and confers water
solubility on the resulting detergent-protein complex. Removing the detergents from the detergent-protein complexes usually leads to the formation
of amorphous precipitates. The aggregation is presumably due to uncovering
of the hydrophobic regions of the intrinsic membrane proteins as detergent
is removed. As shown in Figure 7, however, conditions may be found that
make the isolation of water-soluble and lipid-free intrinsic membrane protein
complexes possible. By mutually covering up the hydrophobic peptide segments of the SFV spike glycoproteins, the proteins can form homodisperse
complexes with a sufficiently polar surface to remain soluble.

E. Transmembrane Location

The question how deep the SFV spike glycoproteins penetrate the lipid bilayer
has been studied using two different experimental approaches [64]. The first
employed the radioactive surface label, ^{35}S-formylmethionyl sulfone methyl-
phosphate [65], and the second the protein cross-linking reagent dimethylsuberimidate [66].

The glycoproteins in intact SFV were caused to react with the surface
label from the outside or both from the inside and the outside using membrane "ghost" preparations (Fig. 5) obtained from the virus by adding enough
Triton X-100 to barely lyse the membrane. When the membrane ghosts were
labeled, the peptide maps of the glycoprotein contained two additional basic,
heavily labeled peptides that were not seen in the peptide maps derived from
the glycoproteins labeled only from the outside (using intact virus). One
possible explanation of this result is that a segment of at least one of the
viral polypeptides extends through the membrane and the two additional peptides seen when labeling was performed from both sides are derived from
those parts of the proteins that are exposed on the inner (nucleocapsid) surface
of the membrane.

The cross-linking experiments confirmed this interpretation. Most of
the SFV glycoproteins were cross-linked to the nucleocapsid when intact
virus particles were treated with dimethylsuberimidate. No cross-linking of
the phospholipids to the nucleocapsid could be detected. As dimethylsuberimidate can maximally bridge a distance of 11 Å, which is about one-fourth
the lipid bilayer thickness in SFV, such extensive cross-linking would be
possible only if the viral glycoproteins lie close to the nucleocapsid, that is,
span the lipid membrane (Fig. 11).

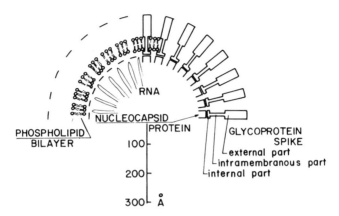

FIG. 11 Proposed structure for the SFV membrane. Taken from
Ref. 106.

The subunit structure of the spikes in the SFV membrane is not fully
settled. Cross-linking experiments with dimethylsuberimidate combined with
Triton X-100 solubilization studies indicated the the SFV spike corresponds
either to a trimer (E1, E2, E3) or to two different structures—separate
dimers of E1 and E2, either of which could contain E3 [67]. On the basis of
available evidence, the former structure appears the more likely. Von Bonsdorff and Harrison have recently demonstrated that the spike glycoproteins
of Sindbis virus (another alphavirus) form a regular icosahedral lattice (T=4)
on the virus surface, probably induced by a similar icosahedral design of
the underlying nucleocapsid [68]. This is in keeping with the structural model
of alphaviruses shown in Figure 11, where the spike proteins, it is assumed,
bind to the nucleocapsid protein in a one-to-one binding ratio. The four polypeptides E1, E2, E3, and the nucleocapsid protein are present in equimolar
amounts in the virus particle.

In this context, lowering the pH to about 6, or glutaraldehyde fixation,
has been observed to cause a contraction of the SFV particle with a decrease
in diameter of about 100 Å [7]. This effect has been studied by Kääriäinen
and coworkers and it appears to be due to a size decrease of the nucleocapsid
[69]. The viral membrane apparently adheres to the nucleocapsid during the
contraction and excess membrane is extruded from the contracted virus
particle into blebs. Spikes are not seen on the surface of these blebs, suggesting that these are mainly formed by viral lipids and that the viral spike
glycoproteins remain bound to the nucleocapsid.

The structure of that part of the protein spikes penetrating the lipid
bilayer is not known, but the available data indicate that the volume occupied
by protein in the bilayer is not very large. If both the polypeptides E1 and E2
spanned the membrane in alpha-helical form [70], less than 15% of the area
in the middle of the bilayer would be occupied by protein. So that even if the

protein : lipid ratio is as high as 3 : 2 in the SFV membrane, most of the
protein is located outside the bilayer (Fig. 11).

IV. BIOSYNTHESIS OF SFV MEMBRANE PROTEINS

When SFV infects an animal cell, the incoming virus takes over the cellular
protein-synthesizing machinery and within three hours almost only virus
proteins are being made. These can therefore be labeled and easily followed
in pulse-chase experiments. Furthermore, through the work of Burge and
Pfefferkorn [71] and others [72-75], a number of temperature-sensitive RNA[+]
mutants of both SFV and Sindbis virus are available, which are blocked in
virus assembly.

All the structural proteins of the virus are translated as one precursor
polyprotein having an apparent molecular weight of about 1.3×10^5 in SDS
gels [76-77]. This has been shown mainly by using temperature-sensitive
mutants. Studies both in vivo and in vitro suggest that the nucleocapsid protein is located at the N-terminal end of this polyprotein [78-80]. Other
mutants have been found where two other precursor proteins can be isolated,
one having a molecular weight about 9.7×10^4 and containing E1 and E2 segments as shown by peptide mapping, and another with a molecular weight
about 8.7×10^4 and containing the nucleocapsid protein and E2 [76, 81-82].
In wild-type infection and in a number of mutants, an additional smaller precursor protein is found with an apparent molecular weight of 6.2×10^4, containing both E2 and E3 [76, 83]. This evidence thus suggests that the order
of the structural proteins in the precursor polyprotein is nucleocapsid
protein-E3 and E2-E1. The nucleocapsid protein is probably first cleaved
from the nascent polyprotein chain and then rapidly bound to the viral RNA
to form the nucleocapsid in the cytoplasm [84-85]. The remaining part of the
polyprotein forming the virus spike is bound to the endoplasmic reticulum
immediately after synthesis and from there transferred membrane-bound to
the cell surface. Whether the polyprotein is translated on cytoplasmic or
membrane-bound ribosomes is not known yet. Cytoplasmic proteins like the
nucleocapsid protein are usually translated on cytoplasmic ribosomes, whereas
the ribosome location used by membrane proteins is still not settled [86]. It
is usually assumed that membrane proteins are made on membrane-bound
ribosomes, but Bretscher [87] has argued that cytoplasmic ribosomes may
be used too. Membrane proteins located towards the cytoplasm may indeed
use the latter type [88-89] but whether this applies also to the intrinsic membrane glycoproteins situated on the external side of the plasma membrane
remains to be seen. Support for a membrane-bound polysome location for
the latter protein class is provided by the fact that the spike glycoproteins of
another virus budding from the plasma membrane, vesicular stomatitis virus,
have recently been found to be made on membrane-bound ribosomes [90-91].
One could perhaps envisage the N-terminal part of the alphavirus polyprotein
being read on a cytoplasmic ribosome until the nucleocapsid polypeptide has

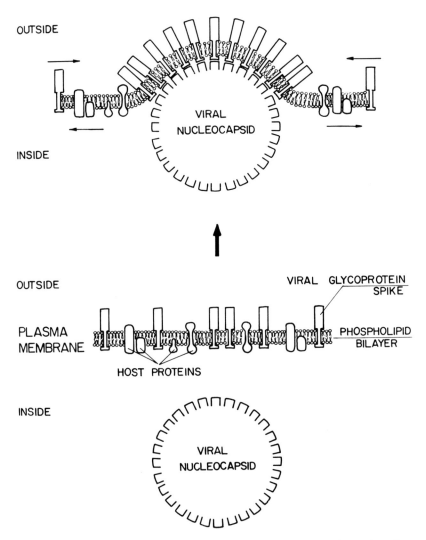

FIG. 12 A hypothetical scheme for the budding of SFV from the plasma membrane of the animal host cell. Taken from Ref. 107.

been cleaved off [8]. The ribosome then becomes bound to the endoplasmic reticulum by means of the exposed N-terminal portion of the (E3, E2, E1) part of the elongating polyprotein. This type of membrane attachment would be essentially transient, limited to a single round of translation for each site of attachment. This question is probably closely related to the next steps in the biosynthesis of the virus membrane: How do the hydrophilic parts of the spike proteins pass through the membrane of the endoplasmic reticulum to the cisternal side to reach the host enzymes involved in glycosylation? Is the next cleavage to occur (that between E1 and E3-E2) taking place at this stage? The mechanism of transport of the spike proteins from the site of synthesis to their destination at the cell surface is another enigma. What is the role of glycosylation? Are the proteins using a pathway similar to that used by the proteins destined for export, or is there a separate route for membrane proteins? The last cleavage is between E2 and E3. The E2-E3 cleavage requires considerably more time than the other two and probably occurs immediately before the budding [8, 9, 92].

The virus spike proteins arrive at the plasma membrane within thirty minutes of their synthesis [85]. Birdwell and Strauss [93] have shown that the first virus glycoproteins arrive at the surface of a chick fibroblast at two hours after infection; the concentration of virus proteins at the surface increases throughout the infection cycle, reaching its maximum by six to eight hours after infection, when virus is budding out at a maximal rate. By three hours after infection, the concentration of virus glycoproteins is sufficient to show plasma membrane modification detected by hemadsorption [94], agglutinability by concavalin A [95], and superinfection exclusion [96]. Several observations indicate that the nucleocapsid is attached to the plasma membrane after the viral spike proteins have been transferred to the membrane [6]. If the viral glycoproteins traverse the plasma membrane, the nucleocapsid may simply link to those parts of the spike proteins that are exposed on the cytoplasmic surface of the host cell membrane [64]. The membrane-bound nucleocapsid could then act as a nucleation site for additional glycoproteins moving into the growing patch by lateral diffusion [93]. Host membrane proteins that have no affinity for the nucleocapsid might move out of the growing patch for steric reasons. The association of the viral spikes with the nucleocapsid proceeds until all binding sites are filled and a mature virus particle is finally released into the extracellular fluid, with the free energy for the budding supplied by the nucleocapsid-spike glycoprotein interactions. The final stage in virus assembly would, according to this view, be due to self-assembly.

Two groups of temperature-sensitive virus mutants have some bearing on the budding. The only mutant so far found in complementation group E produces both nucleocapsids and a functional hemagglutinating E1 polypeptide at the nonpermissive temperature [97]. The nucleocapsids line up under the plasma membrane, but no budding occurs at 40 °C [98]. Neither does the cleavage between E2 and E3 take place [99]. The exact defect is not known, but this mutant group is thought to be defective in the E2 or E3 region. Mutants in group D have a defect in the hemagglutinating polypeptide E1 [8]. In cells infected with these mutants at the nonpermissive temperature, no functional E1 appears to be inserted into the plasma membrane and in this case the nucleocapsids are found dispersed throughout the cytoplasm [98]. These findings suggest that a functional E1 polypeptide is essential for the binding of the nucleocapsids to the surface membrane. It will be interesting to correlate the molecular defects involved with the detailed structure of the alphavirus spike glycoprotein.

ACKNOWLEDGMENTS

We wish to thank our colleagues in Helsinki, especially Drs. Kääriäinen and Renkonen for valuable help and inspiring discussions. We are also grateful to Drs. S. Schlesinger, and E. G. and J. H. Strauss for communicating material to us before publication. Most of our own experimental work has been done at the Department of Serology and Bacteriology, University of Helsinki, Finland, and has been supported by grants from the National Research Council for Medical Sciences and the Sigrid Juselius Foundation, Finland.

REFERENCES

1. J. Lenard and R. W. Compans, Biochim. Biophys. Acta, 344, 51 (1974).
2. H.-D. Klenk, Current Topics in Microbiology and Immunology, 68, 29 (1974).
3. R. M. Franklin, Current Topics in Microbiology and Immunology, 68, 108 (1974).
4. H. Fraenkel-Conrat and R. R. Wagner, eds., Comprehensive Virology. New York: Plenum Press, 1974.
5. M. C. Horzinek, J. Gen. Virol., 20, 87 (1973).
6. E. R. Pfefferkorn and D. Shapiro, Comprehensive Virology, Vol. 2, ed. H. Fraenkel-Conrat and R. R. Wagner. New York: Plenum Press, 1974, pp. 171-230.
7. C.-H. von Bonsdorff, Commentationes Biologiae Societas Scientarum Fennica, 74, 1 (1973).
8. J. H. Strauss and E. G. Strauss, in Molecular Biology of Animal Viruses, ed. D. Nayak. New York: Marcel Dekker, in press.
9. K. Simons and L. Kääriäinen, Biochem. Biophys. Res. Commun., 38, 981 (1970).

10. S. C. Harrison, A. David, J. Jumblatt, and J. E. Darnell, Jr., J. Mol. Biol., 60, 523 (1971).
11. J. H. Strauss, B. W. Burge, and J. E. Darnell, Jr., Virology, 37, 367 (1969).
12. M. Mussgay, P.-J. Enzmann, and J. Horst, Arch. Ges. Virusforschg., 31, 81 (1970).
13. N. H. Acheson and I. Tamm, Virology, 32, 128 (1967).
14. M. W. Davey, D. P. Dennett, and L. Dalgarno, J. Gen. Virol., 20, 225 (1973).
15. J. R. Gliedman, J. F. Smith, and D. T. Brown, J. Virol., 16, 913 (1975).
16. R. Laine, H. Söderlund, and O. Renkonen, Intervirology, 1, 110 (1973).
17. O. Renkonen, L. Kääriäinen, K. Simons, and C. G. Gahmberg, Virology, 46, 318 (1971).
18. J. P. Quigley, D. B. Rifkin, and E. Reich, Virology, 46, 106 (1971).
19. C. B. Hirschberg and P. W. Robbins, Virology, 61, 602 (1974).
20. O. Renkonen, A. Luukkonen, J. Brotherus, and L. Kääriäinen, Control of Proliferation in Animal Cells, ed. B. Clarkson and R. Baserga. New York: Cold Spring Harbor Laboratory, 1974, pp. 495-504.
21. E. R. Pfefferkorn and R. L. Clifford, Virology, 23, 217 (1964).
22. H. Garoff, K. Simons, and O. Renkonen, Virology, 61, 493 (1974).
23. R. W. Compans, Nature New Biol., 229, 114 (1971).
24. C. G. Gahmberg, G. Utermann, and K. Simons, FEBS Letters, 28, 179 (1972).
25. D. H. Clarke and J. Casals, Amer. J. Trop. Med. Hyg., 7, 561 (1958).
26. A. Helenius and K. Simons, Biochim. Biophys. Acta, 415, 29 (1975).
27. R. Becker, A. Helenius, and K. Simons, Biochemistry, 14, 1835 (1975).
28. A. Helenius and H. Söderlund, Biochim. Biophys. Acta, 307, 287 (1973).
29. K. Simons, A. Helenius, and H. Garoff, J. Mol. Biol., 80, 119 (1973).
30. A. Helenius, E. Fries, H. Garoff, and K. Simons, Biochim. Biophys. Acta, 436, 319 (1976).
31. H. Nakayama, K. Shinoda, and E. Hutchinson, J. Phys. Chem., 70, 3502 (1966).
32. B. Moss and E. N. Rosenblum, J. Biol. Chem., 247, 5194 (1972).
33. A. Tzagoloff and H. S. Penefsky, Methods of Enzymology, Vol. 22, ed. W. B. Jakoby. New York: Academic Press, 1971, pp. 219-230.
34. C. Tanford, Advan. Prot. Chem., 23, 211 (1968).
35. A. Helenius and K. Simons, J. Biol. Chem., 247, 3656 (1972).
36. S. Makino, J. A. Reynolds, and C. Tanford, J. Biol. Chem., 248, 4926 (1973).
37. R. Pitt-Rivers and F. S. A. Impiombato, Biochem. J., 109, 825 (1968).
38. C. A. Schnaitman, Arch. Biochem. Biophys., 157, 553 (1973).
39. L. Spatz and P. Strittmatter, J. Biol. Chem., 248, 793 (1973).
40. S. P. Grefrath and J. A. Reynolds, Proc. Nat. Acad. Sci. U.S., 71, 3913 (1974).

41. C. Tanford, Y. Nozaki, J. A. Reynolds, and S. Makino, Biochemistry, 13, 2369 (1974).
42. R. A. Capaldi and G. Vanderkooi, Proc. Nat. Acad. Sci. U.S., 69, 930 (1972).
43. K. Mattila, A. Luukkanen, and O. Renkonen, Biochim. Biophys. Acta, 419, 435 (1976).
44. B. M. Sefton and K. Keegstra, J. Virol., 14, 522 (1974).
45. S. Schlesinger, C. Gottlieb, P. Feil, N. Gelb, and S. Kornfeld, J. Virol., 17, 239 (1976).
46. S. A. Moyer and D. F. Summers, Cell, 70, 63 (1974).
47. G. Utermann and K. Simons, J. Mol. Biol., 85, 560 (1974).
48. A. Ito and R. Sato, J. Biol. Chem., 243, 4922 (1968).
49. L. Spatz and P. Strittmatter, Proc. Nat. Acad. Sci. U.S., 68, 1042 (1971).
50. J. P. Segrest, R. L. Jackson, V. T. Marchesi, R. B. Guyer, and W. Terry, Biochem. Biophys. Res. Commun., 49, 964 (1972).
51. W. G. Laver, Adv. Virus Res., 18, 57 (1973).
52. R. H. Schloemer and R. R. Wagner, J. Virol., 16, 237 (1975).
53. D. A. Marvin and E. J. Wachtel, Nature, 253, 19 (1975).
54. S. Maroux, D. Louvard, Biochim. Biophys. Acta (1975), in press.
55. H. Sigrist, P. Bonner, and G. Semenza, Biochim. Biophys. Acta, 406, 433 (1975).
56. M. S. Bretscher, Nature New Biol., 231, 229 (1971).
57. H. C. Berg and D. Hirsh, Anal. Biochem., 66, 629 (1975).
58. K. Weber and D. J. Kuter, J. Biol. Chem., 246, 4504 (1971).
59. R. A. Laskey and A. D. Mills, Eur. J. Biochem., 56, 335 (1975).
60. M. T. Laico, E. Ruoslahti, D. S. Papermaster, and W. J. Dreyer, Proc. Nat. Acad. Sci. U.S., 67, 120 (1970).
61. W. J. Dreyer, D. S. Papermaster, and H. Kühn, Ann. N.Y. Acad. Sci., 195, 61 (1972).
62. J. J. Holland, M. Doyle, J. Perrault, D. T. Kingsbury, and J. Etchinson, Biochem. Biophys. Res. Commun., 46, 634 (1972).
63. N. C. Robinson and C. Tanford, Biochemistry, 14, 369 (1975).
64. H. Garoff and K. Simons, Proc. Nat. Acad. Sci. U.S., 71, 3988 (1974).
65. M. S. Bretscher, J. Mol. Biol., 58, 775 (1971).
66. G. E. Davies and G. R. Stark, Proc. Nat. Acad. Sci. U.S., 66, 651 (1970).
67. H. Garoff, Virology, 62, 385 (1974).
68. C.-H. von Bonsdorff and S. C. Harrison, J. Virol., 16, 141 (1975).
69. H. Söderlund, L. Kääriäinen, C.-H. von Bonsdorff, and P. Weckström, Virology, 47, 753 (1972).
70. R. Henderson and P. N. T. Unwin, Nature, 257, 28 (1975).
71. B. W. Burge and E. R. Pfefferkorn, Virology, 30, 204 (1966).
72. S. Keränen and L. Kääriäinen, Acta Path. Microbiol., Scand. sect. B., 82, 810 (1974).

73. E. G. Strauss, E. M. Lenches, and J. H. Strauss, Virology, 74, 154 (1976).
74. G. J. Atkins, J. Samuels, and S. I. T. Kennedy, J. Gen. Virol., 25, 371 (1974).
75. K. B. Tan, J. F. Sambrook, and A. J. D. Bellett, Virology, 38, 427 (1969).
76. M. J. Schlesinger and S. Schlesinger, J. Virol., 11, 1013 (1973).
77. S. Keränen and L. Kääriäinen, J. Virol., 16, 388 (1975).
78. J. C. S. Clegg, Nature, 254, 454 (1975).
79. S. Schlesinger and M. J. Schlesinger, J. Virol., 10, 925 (1972).
80. N. Glanville, J. Morser, P. Uomala, and L. Kääriäinen, Eur. J. Biochem., 64, 167 (1976).
81. D. T. Simmons and J. H. Strauss, J. Mol. Biol., 86, 397 (1974).
82. B.-E. Lachmi, N. Glanville, S. Keränen, and L. Kääriäinen, J. Virol., 16, 1615 (1975).
83. K. Simons, S. Keränen, and L. Kääriäinen, FEBS Letters, 29, 87 (1973).
84. H. Söderlund, Intervirology, 1, 354 (1973).
85. C. M. Scheele and E. R. Pfefferkorn, J. Virol., 3, 369 (1969).
86. G. Palade, Science, 189, 347 (1975).
87. M. S. Bretscher, Science, 181, 622 (1973).
88. D. Lowe and T. Hallinan, Biochem. J., 136, 825 (1973).
89. H. F. Lodish and B. Small, J. Cell Biol., 65, 51 (1975).
90. M. J. Grubman, S. A. Moyer, A. K. Banerjee, and E. Ehrenfeld, Biochem. Biophys. Res. Commun., 62, 531 (1975).
91. T. G. Morrison and H. F. Lodish, J. Biol. Chem., 250, 6955 (1975).
92. B. M. Sefton, G. G. Wickus, and B. W. Burge, J. Virol., 11, 730 (1973).
93. C. R. Birdwell and J. H. Strauss, J. Virol., 14, 366 (1974).
94. B. W. Burge and E. R. Pfefferkorn, J. Virol., 1, 956 (1967).
95. C. R. Birdwell and J. H. Strauss, J. Virol., 11, 502 (1973).
96. J. S. Pierce, E. G. Strauss, and J. H. Strauss, J. Virol., 13, 1030 (1974).
97. B. W. Burge and E. R. Pfefferkorn, J. Mol. Biol., 35, 193 (1968).
98. D. T. Brown and J. E. Smith, J. Virol., 15, 1262 (1975).
99. K. J. Jones, M. R. F. Waite, and H. R. Bose, J. Virol., 13, 809 (1974).
100. J. C. Meunier, R. W. Olsen, and J. P. Changeux, FEBS Letters, 24, 63 (1972).
101. M. S. Rubin and A. Tzagoloff, J. Biol. Chem., 248, 4269 (1973).
102. H. Walter and W. Hasselbach, Eur. J. Biochem., 36, 110 (1973).
103. B. H. Osborn, C. Sardet, and A. Helenius, Eur. J. Biochem., 44, 383 (1974).
104. S. Clarke, J. Biol. Chem., 250, 5459 (1975).
105. A. Helenius and C.-H. von Bonsdorff, Biochim. Biophys. Acta, 436, 895 (1976).

106. K. Simons, H. Garoff, and A. Helenius, 10th FEBS Meeting. Amster-
     dam: North-Holland Publishing Co., 1975, pp. 35-91.
107. H. Garoff and K. Simons, in Cell Membranes and Viral Envelopes,
     ed. H. A. Blough and J. M. Tiffany. New York: Academic Press, in
     press.
108. D. M. Neville, Jr., J. Biol. Chem., 246, 6328 (1971).
109. K. Weber and M. Osborn, J. Biol. Chem., 244, 4406 (1969).

Numbers in parentheses are reference numbers and indicate that an author's work is referred to although his name is not cited in the text. Underlined numbers give the page on which the complete reference is listed.